Sports Injuries of the Elbow

Adam C. Watts · Lennard Funk
Michael Hayton · Chye Yew Ng
Mike Walton

Editors

Sports Injuries of the Elbow

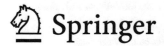 Springer

Editors
Adam C. Watts
Wrightington Hospital
Wigan
UK

Lennard Funk
Wrightington Hospital
Wigan
UK

Michael Hayton
Wrightington Hospital
Wigan
UK

Chye Yew Ng
Wrightington Hospital
Wigan
UK

Mike Walton
Wrightington Hospital
Wigan
UK

ISBN 978-3-030-52381-7   ISBN 978-3-030-52379-4   (eBook)
https://doi.org/10.1007/978-3-030-52379-4

This Springer imprint is published by the registered company Springer Nature Switzerland AG
The registered company address is: Gewerbestrasse 11, 6330 Cham, Switzerland

Contents

Clinical Anatomy of the Elbow

1

James R. A. Smith and Rouin Amirfeyz

Contents

J. R. A. Smith
Severn Deanery, Bristol, UK

R. Amirfeyz (✉)
Bristol Royal Infirmary, Bristol, UK
e-mail: rouin.amirfeyz@uhbristol.nhs.uk

© The Editor(s) (if applicable) and The Author(s), under exclusive license to Springer Nature
Switzerland AG 2021
A. C. Watts et al. (eds.), *Sports Injuries of the Elbow*, https://doi.org/10.1007/978-3-030-52379-4_1

Key Learning Points

1. The elbow joint is comprised of three articulations; the humeroulnar, radiocapitellar and proximal radioulnar joints.
2. The articulations are surrounded buy a joint capsule with condensations that form the lateral ligament complex and medial collateral ligament.
3. Three important nerves cross the elbow joint; the ulnar nerve, median nerve and radial nerve.
4. The elbow is supplied by the brachial, radial and ulnar arteries and their recurrent branches. The radial head is intracapsular and relies on retrograde blood flow.

1.1   Introduction

A thorough understanding of the anatomical structures is fundamental to correct diagnosis and safe treatment of disorders of the elbow. This chapter provides an overview of the surgical anatomy, and is divided into four anatomical sections: osteoarticular, capsuloligamentous, muscular and neurovascular.

1.2   Osteoarticular Anatomy

The elbow joint is comprised of three articulations: the humeroulnar, radiocapitellar and proximal radioulnar joints (although located within the capsule of the elbow joint this is really a part of the forearm joint).

1.2.1   The Humerus

The humerus terminates distally as a medial and lateral column, each forming a condyle and an epicondyle. These two columns hold the trochlea and the capitellum. The trochlea is an asymmetrical spool-shaped surface that articulates with

the greater sigmoid notch of the olecranon. Its medial aspect projects further distally. The capitellum is hemispherical in shape and articulates with the concave surfaced radial head. The trochlear groove separates the two articular surfaces (Fig. 1.1).

The trochlear-capitellar articular surface is internally rotated approximately 5–7° in relation to the epicondylar axis [1]. Additionally, this surface has a valgus angle of between 6 and 8° when compared to the long axis of the humerus [2]. This is an important issue when the joint axis of rotation is to be surgically reproduced (fixation of fracture or application of a dynamic external fixator). In the sagittal plane the articular surface of the humerus protrudes approximately 30° anterior to the long axis of the humerus.

On the anterior surface of the humerus, proximal to the articular surface, lie the coronoid and radial fossae. These accommodate the coronoid process and radial head when the elbow is in full flexion. Similarly, on the posterior aspect of the humerus, the olecranon fossa accommodates the olecranon process of the ulna, permitting full extension of the elbow. The normal range of elbow flexion/extension is approximately 0–150°, with 30–130° necessary to maintain a functional arc [3]. A sulcus, posterior to the medial epicondyle, accommodates the passage of the ulna nerve (Fig. 1.2).

1.2.2   The Ulna

The main articulating portion of the proximal ulna is the greater sigmoid (or trochlear) notch. It is formed predominantly by the olecranon, with the coronoid process extending the joint surface anteriorly (Fig. 1.3). It is elliptical in shape, with a longitudinal ridge conveying a stable and congruent articulation with the trochlea, forming the humeroulnar joint. It is oriented approximately 30° posterior to the long axis of the ulna to match the anterior angulation of the distal humerus. The coronoid process is comprised of a large antero-

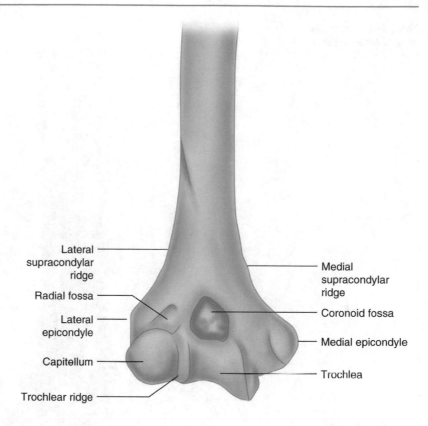

Fig. 1.1 Anterior view
of right distal humerus

Lateral supracondylar ridge

Radial fossa

Lateral epicondyle

Capitellum

Trochlear ridge

Medial supracondylar ridge

Coronoid fossa

Medial epicondyle

Trochlea

medial facet and smaller anterolateral facet that articulate with the medial trochlea and lateral trochlea respectively.

The articular cartilage surface of the trochlear notch is interrupted by a variable transverse 'bare area' of bone, located midway between the tip of the olecranon and the coronoid process (Fig. 1.4).

Distal to the trochlear notch, on the lateral aspect of the coronoid process, lies the lesser sigmoid (or radial) notch. This accommodates the radial head, forming the proximal radioulnar joint. The supinator crest originates at the distal part of the lesser sigmoid notch, and provides the origin of the supinator muscle and on the most proximal part of it, the insertion for the lateral ulnar collateral ligament (LUCL).

On the medial coronoid, lies an important bony prominence—the sublime tubercle. This provides the insertion site for the anterior bundle of the anterior medial collateral ligament

(AMCL), and is fundamental to both the valgus stability of the elbow (see capsuloligamentous anatomy section) and maintaining the trochlea within the greater sigmoid notch.

1.2.3   The Radius

The surface of the radial head is concave in shape. Both the proximal end and approximately its circumference are covered with articular cartilage, allowing a smooth articulation with both the capitellum, and the lesser sigmoid notch. The radial neck constitutes the most distal intra-articular portion of the proximal radius.

On the anteromedial surface of the radius, just distal to the neck, lays the bicipital tuberosity. This is the point of insertion for the biceps brachii tendon.

Fig. 1.2 Posterior view
of right distal humerus

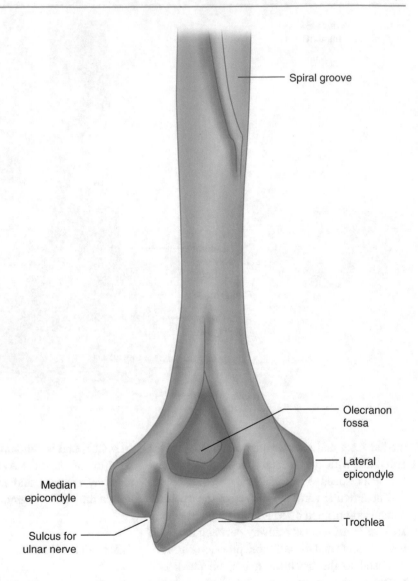

Spiral groove

Olecranon
fossa

Lateral
epicondyle

Median
epicondyle

Trochlea

Sulcus for
ulnar nerve

1.3   Capsuloligamentous
         Anatomy

1.3.1   Joint Capsule

The three elbow articulations are surrounded by
a joint capsule and form a synovial joint. The
anterior capsule inserts proximally above the
radial and coronoid fossae of the humerus, and
attaches to the anterior surface of the coronoid

medially (sparing the tip, which remains intra-
articular) and the annular ligament laterally.
Posteriorly it attaches above the olecranon fossa
and around the medial and lateral margins of the
sigmoid notch.

The maximum capacity of the capsule is
25–30 mL at approximately 80° of flexion [4].
The capsule is innervated by the nerves that cross
it; namely the musculocutaneous, radial, median
and ulnar nerves.

Fig. 1.3 Lateral view of
right proximal ulna

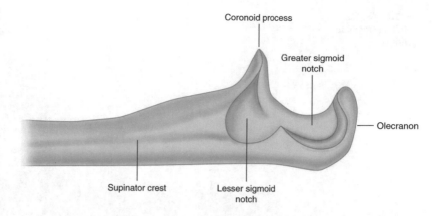

Fig. 1.4 Right proximal
radioulnar joint

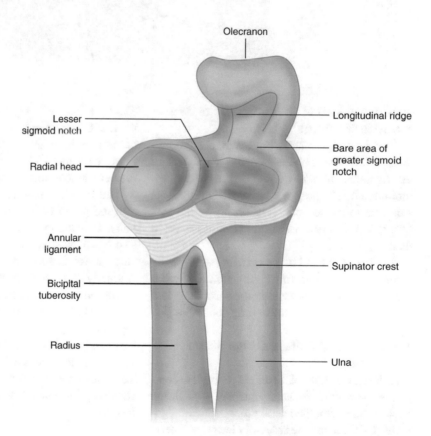

1.3.2   Ligaments

1.3.2.1 Medial Collateral
Ligament Complex

The medial collateral ligament comprises an
anterior and posterior bundle, and a supporting
transverse ligament; the function of which is not
well understood (Fig. 1.5).

The anterior bundle originates from the
anteroinferior aspect of the medial epicondyle
[5], and inserts on the sublime tubercle of the
ulna, on average 18 mm posterior from the tip
of the coronoid [6]. The centre of the anterior
bundle origin lies at the axis of rotation of the
elbow [7, 8], however, it is comprised of an anterior and posterior band, which are maximally

Fig. 1.5 Medial
collateral ligament
complex

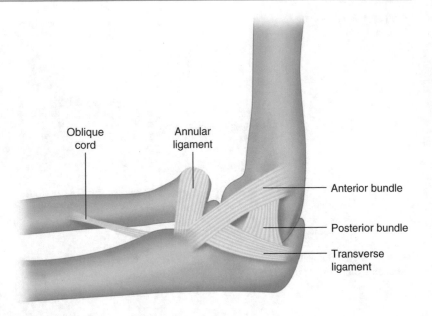

tight (functional) at different ranges of flexion-extension arc [9, 10].

The posterior bundle originates posterior to the anterior bundle on the medial epicondyle, and inserts along the mid-portion of the greater sigmoid notch. The posterior bundle is lax in extension due to its posterior relationship to the axis of rotation. It, therefore, restrains valgus stress in flexion only [8, 10].

The anterior band of the anterior bundle is the primary constraint to valgus and internal rotatory forces. The posterior band is the secondary, and the posterior bundle is the tertiary constraint [9].

1.3.2.2 Lateral Collateral Ligament Complex

The lateral collateral ligament complex comprises the radial collateral ligament (RCL), the annular ligament, the lateral ulnar collateral ligament (LUCL), and the accessory lateral collateral ligament (ALCL) (when it exists) (Fig. 1.6).

The RCL and LUCL both originate from the centre of rotation on the lateral epicondyle, and thus are isometric throughout elbow flexion [11].

The RCL inserts along the annular ligament and the LUCL inserts onto the tubercle of the supinator crest of the ulna. Both ligaments resist varus stress, with the LUCL fundamental to holding the greater sigmoid notch onto the trochlea [12].

The annular ligament attaches to the anterior and posterior margins of the lesser sigmoid notch, maintaining the proximal radioulnar joint. The ALCL stabilises the annular ligament during varus stress of the elbow but sometimes it is not distinctly different from the capsule of the joint.

Recent evidence suggests a fifth element, the posterolateral or Osborn-Cotterill ligament arising from the posterolateral aspect of the capitellum and inserting in to the margin of the greater sigmoid notch proximal to the supinator crest. This has been shown to contribute to posterior stability of the radial head at around 60° elbow flexion.

1.4 Muscular Anatomy

Muscular anatomy is summarised in Table 1.1

Fig. 1.6 Lateral collateral ligament complex

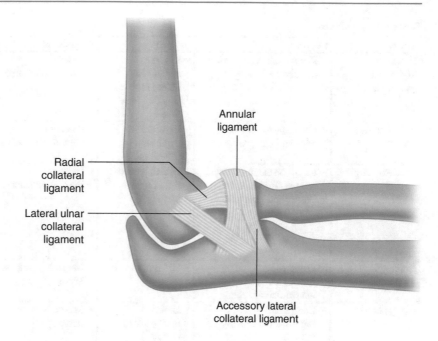

Annular
ligament

Radial
collateral
ligament

Lateral ulnar
collateral
ligament

Accessory lateral
collateral ligament

Table 1.1 Details the muscles that act upon or cross the elbow joint

Muscle	Origin	Insertion	Innervation	Action
Triceps brachii	• Long head—infraglenoid tubercle of scapula • Lateral head—superior to spiral groove of humerus • Medial head—inferior to spiral groove of humerus	• Olecranon • Additional attachment to dorsal fascia of forearm	• Radial nerve • Axillary nerve recognised variation for long head [13]	• Elbow extension
Anconeus	• Posterior lateral epicondyle	• Lateral posterior proximal ulna	• Radial nerve	• Elbow extension and stabilisation
Supinator	• Anterior lateral epicondyle • Lateral collateral ligament complex • Supinator crest of proximal ulna	• Lateral proximal radial diaphysis	• Posterior interosseous nerve	• Forearm supination
Brachioradialis	• Lateral supracondylar ridge of humerus • Lateral intermuscular septum	• Radial styloid	• Radial nerve	• Elbow flexion • Forearm pro- and supination
Extensor carpii radialis longus	• Lateral supracondylar ridge of humerus • Lateral intermuscular septum • Common extensor origin of lateral epicondyle	• Dorsal, radial surface of index finger metacarpal	• Radial nerve	• Wrist extension and radial deviation
Extensor carpii radialis brevis	• Common extensor origin of lateral epicondyle • Radial collateral ligament	• Dorsal surface of middle finger metacarpal	• Posterior interosseous nerve	• Wrist extension

(continued)

Table 1.1 (continued)

Muscle	Origin	Insertion	Innervation	Action
Extensor digitorum communis	• Common extensor origin of lateral epicondyle	• Extensor expansions of index, middle, ring and little fingers	• Posterior interosseous nerve	• PIPJ/DIPJ of Fingers (and wrist) extension
Extensor digiti minimi	• Common extensor origin of lateral epicondyle	• Extensor expansion of little finger	• Posterior interosseous nerve	• Little finger PIPJ/DIPJ extension
Extensor carpii ulnaris	• Common extensor origin of lateral epicondyle • Posterior aspect of ulna	• Dorsal base of little finger metacarpal	• Posterior interosseous nerve	• Wrist extension • Ulnar deviation of wrist • Dynamic stabiliser of distal radioulnar joint
Brachialis	• Distal anterior humerus • Lateral and medial intermuscular septum	• Ulnar tuberosity	• Musculocutaneous nerve	• Elbow flexion
Biceps brachii	• Long head—supraglenoid tubercle of scapula • Short head—coracoid process	• Bicipital tuberosity of radius	• Musculocutaneous nerve	• Forearm supination • Elbow flexion
Flexor carpi ulnaris	• Humeral head—common flexor origin of medial epicondyle • Ulnar head—medial olecranon	• Base of little finger metacarpal via the pisiform and hamate	• Ulnar nerve	• Wrist flexion • Ulnar deviation of wrist
Flexor digitorum superficialis	• Humeroulnar head—common flexor origin of medial epicondyle, medial collateral ligament and the medial side of the coronoid • Radial head—anterior radial aspect	• Volar middle phalanges of index, middle, ring and little fingers	• Median nerve	• Finger flexion at proximal interphalangeal joint
Palmaris longus	• Common flexor origin of medial epicondyle	• Palmar aponeurosis	• Median nerve	• Wrist flexion
Flexor carpi radialis	• Common flexor origin of medial epicondyle	• Volar base of index finger metacarpal	• Median nerve	• Wrist flexion • Radial deviation of wrist
Pronator teres	• Humeral head—common flexor origin of medial epicondyle • Ulnar head—coronoid process	• Radial surface of midshaft radius just distal to insertion of supinator	• Median nerve	• Forearm pronation • Elbow flexion

1.5 Neurovascular Anatomy

1.5.1 Radial Nerve

The radial nerve is derived from the C5-T1 nerve roots, and is a terminal branch of the posterior cord of the brachial plexus. It exits the axilla through the lateral triangular space (teres major superiorly, long head of triceps medially, humerus laterally) accompanied by the profunda brachii artery, and passes into the posterior compartment of the arm. It winds around the humerus over the spiral (or radial) groove, to appear on the lateral aspect of the humerus, where it pierces the lateral intermuscular septum to enter the anterior compartment of the arm. It then approaches the elbow between the brachialis and brachioradialis muscles. It is readily identified 1–2 cm proximal to the medial tip of triceps aponeurosis as an intraoperative landmark. Its course, interestingly, follows the superior border of the aponeurosis coming out of intermuscular septum 1–2 cm proximal to the lateral tip of aponeurosis [14].

The radial nerve then passes under the cover of extensor carpi radialis longus and brevis, and emerges anterior to the lateral epicondyle. At the level of the radiocapitellar joint, it divides into the superficial radial and posterior interosseous nerves.

The superficial radial nerve continues distally in the forearm under the brachioradialis muscle towards the wrist. The posterior interosseous nerve passes between the two heads of supinator to enter the posterior compartment of the forearm. The proximity of the nerve to the proximal radius is dependent on rotational position of the forearm [15], where the nerve is more proximal and under tension in full supination and relaxed and 'away' in pronation.

Damage to the radial nerve most commonly occurs following fractures of the humeral shaft or the proximal radius.

1.5.2 Median Nerve

The median nerve is derived from the C6-T1 nerve roots, and is a terminal branch of both the medial and lateral cords of the brachial plexus. It leaves the axilla at the inferior margin of teres major. It descends in the anterior compartment of the arm between the biceps brachii and brachialis muscles, in association with the brachial artery. In the upper arm it lies lateral to the artery, but crosses over in the mid-arm to lie medial to it. The artery and nerve then pass deep to the bicipital aponeurosis at the elbow, lying medial to the biceps brachii tendon and anterior to the brachialis muscle.

The nerve then passes under the humeral head of pronator teres, and between the humeroulnar and radial heads of the flexor digitorum superficialis muscle to continue distally in the anterior compartment of the forearm. The median nerve gives off the anterior interosseous nerve in the forearm between 5 and 8 cm distal to the level of the lateral epicondyle, usually immediately distal to the humeral head of pronator teres [16].

1.5.3 Ulnar Nerve

The ulnar nerve is the largest branch of the medial cord of the brachial plexus, with nerve roots originating from spinal levels C8-T1. It exits the axilla between the axillary nerve and vein, and descends medial to the brachial artery.

Half-way down the arm it pierces the medial intermuscular septum to lie on the posteromedial aspect of the humerus. The nerve passes between the medial intermuscular septum (anterior) and the medial head of triceps (posterior), and into the sulcus of the ulna nerve—a depression on the back of the medial epicondyle of the humerus (Fig. 1.2). It then passes into the anterior compartment of the forearm through the cubital tunnel (Fig. 1.7).

The cubital tunnel is approximately 5 cm in length. The medial epicondyle forms the medial wall and base proximally, and the olecranon comprises the lateral wall. A fibrous aponeurosis called Osborne's ligament forms the roof, connecting the medial epicondyle and olecranon proximally, and is continuous with the fascia of the humeral and ulnar heads of flexor carpii ulnaris distally. The floor is comprised of the joint capsule and the medial collateral ligaments.

After passing through the cubital tunnel, the ulna nerve passes between the two heads of flexor carpii ulnaris, and continues in the forearm on the muscle belly of flexor digitorum profundus, beneath the flexor carpii ulnaris muscle.

Fig. 1.7 Cubital tunnel

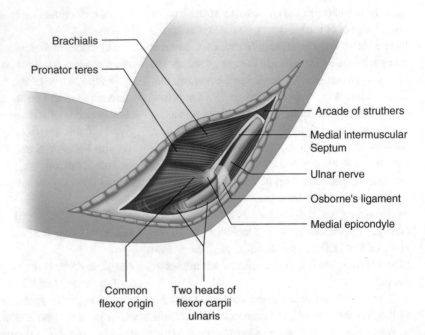

Brachialis

Pronator teres

Arcade of struthers

Medial intermuscular Septum

Ulnar nerve

Osborne's ligament

Medial epicondyle

Common flexor origin

Two heads of flexor carpii ulnaris

1.5.4 Medial Cutaneous Nerves of the Arm and Forearm

The medial cutaneous nerve of the arm is the smallest branch of the medial cord of the brachial plexus. It leaves the axilla posterior to the axillary vein, then passing to its medial side, where it contributes fibres to the intercostobrachial nerve. It descends medial to the brachial artery and pierces the brachial fascia in the middle third of the arm. It provides cutaneous innervation to the medial aspect of the distal third of the arm, extending as far as the elbow.

The medial cutaneous nerve of the forearm also originates from the medial cord of the brachial plexus. It descends the arm with the medial cutaneous nerve, and pierces the brachial fascia with the basilic vein. It divides into an anterior and posterior branch, and passes anterior to the medial epicondyle of the humerus. The anterior branch passes in front of the median basilic vein, and descends on the ulnar side of the forearm. The posterior branch passes obliquely on the medial side of the basilic vein to the posterior aspect of the forearm. It is often encountered during decompression of the ulnar nerve around the cubital tunnel, and injury can lead to pain-

ful neuroma [17]. The nerves provide cutaneous innervation to the anteromedial, medial and posteromedial aspect of the forearm to the level of the wrist.

1.5.5 Lateral Cutaneous Nerves of the Arm and Forearm

The skin of the lateral arm is innervated by the terminal branch of the posterior cord of the axillary nerve (superior lateral cutaneous nerve of the arm), and a branch of the radial nerve (inferior lateral cutaneous nerve of the arm), which supply the superolateral and inferolateral aspects, respectively.

The lateral cutaneous nerve of the forearm is the sensory continuation of the musculocutaneous nerve. The musculocutaneous nerve arises from the lateral cord of the brachial plexus, from nerve roots C5-C7. It passes into the arm in the coracobrachialis muscle, and passes between the biceps brachii and brachialis muscles to the lateral side of the arm. It pierces the brachial fascia lateral to the biceps tendon, to become the lateral cutaneous nerve of the forearm. At the level of cubital crease, it usually lies just lateral to the

Fig. 1.8 Anterior
extraosseous vascular
anatomy

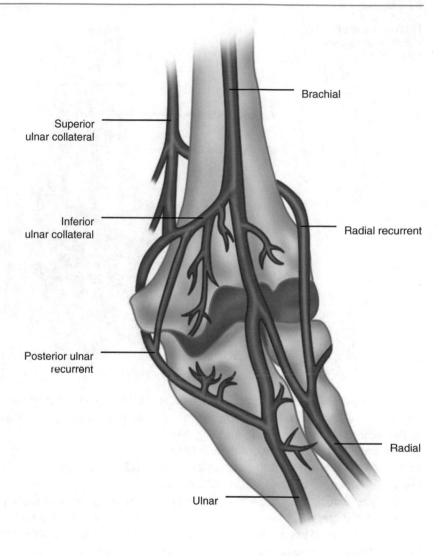

Brachial

Superior
ulnar collateral

Inferior
ulnar collateral

Radial recurrent

Posterior ulnar
recurrent

Radial

Ulnar

cephalic vein. It then passes over the anterolateral aspect of the elbow, and divides into an anterior and posterior branch, innervating the skin of the lateral forearm.

1.5.6 Arteries

The elbow is supplied by the brachial, radial and ulnar arteries and their recurrent branches.

The brachial artery is the continuation of the axillary artery at the inferior border of teres major. At this level it gives off its major branch, the profunda brachii, which passes through the lateral triangular space with the radial nerve towards the

anterolateral elbow. The brachial artery courses the medial arm between the median and ulnar nerves. After passing under the lacertus fibrosus, it enters the antecubital fossa in the midline of the elbow, lying medial to the tendon of biceps brachii. At the level of the radial neck, it bifurcates into the radial and ulnar arteries.

The radial artery runs distally under brachioradialis towards the wrist, medial to the superficial radial nerve. The ulnar artery passes deep towards the anteromedial aspect of the forearm, to lie first upon brachialis and later flexor digitorum profundus as it courses to the wrist.

The collateral supply of the elbow has been described to comprise three arcades: medial,

Fig. 1.9 Posterior
extraosseous vascular
anatomy

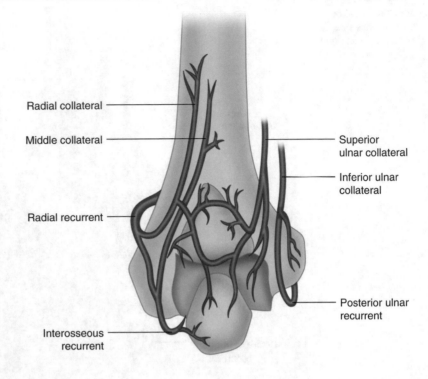

Radial collateral

Middle collateral

Radial recurrent

Interosseous
recurrent

Superior
ulnar collateral

Inferior ulnar
collateral

Posterior ulnar
recurrent

lateral and posterior [18]. The medial arcade is formed by the superior and inferior ulnar collateral branches from the brachial artery, which anastomose the posterior ulnar recurrent branch of the ulnar artery around the medial epicondyle (Fig. 1.8). The medial arcade supplies the medial epicondyle, medial aspect of the trochlea, and the posteromedial olecranon.

The lateral arcade is formed by the descending radial and middle collateral arteries (originating from the profunda brachii), anatomising with the ascending interosseous recurrent and radial recurrent arteries on the posterior aspect of the lateral epicondyle. The lateral arcade supplies the lateral epicondyle and the capitellum.

The posterior arcade is formed in the olecranon fossa by anastomosis of the superior ulnar, radial and middle collateral arteries proximally, and the interosseous recurrent artery distally. The posterior arcade supplies the lateral aspect of the trochlear, the supracondylar region and also branches to the olecranon (Fig. 1.9).

The radial head is intracapsular and receives its blood supply from branches of the recurrent radial artery that pass retrograde up the neck of the radius. The olecranon receives its supply from

the posterior ulnar recurrent and the interosseous recurrent arteries, and from the posterior arcade.

1.5.7 Veins

The deep veins of the upper limb are the venae comitantes of the arteries, ending at the inferior border of teres major, where they are joined by the basilic vein to form the axillary vein.

The major superficial veins are the cephalic and basilic veins, which communicate over the antecubital fossa via the median cubital vein. The cephalic vein drains the lateral upper limb, and joins the axillary vein after piercing the deltopectoral fascia. The basilic vein drains the medial upper limb and pierces the brachial fascia to join the brachial vein in the arm.

Q&A

- What are the important elements of the coronoid process?

  The coronoid process is the primary stabiliser of the elbow joint and is made of two facets, anteromedial and anterolateral, that articulate with the trochlea and also has a medial projection the sublime tubercle into which the anterior band of the medial collateral ligament inserts

- What is the lateral ligament complex?

    The lateral ligament complex is a thickening of the lateral joint capsule that can be considered as five elements that contribute to the stability of the lateral ulnohumeral joint and radial head. The complex arises from the lateral epicondyle and has a primary element, the lateral ulna collateral ligament, that passes to the supinator crest, the radial collateral that inserts to the annular ligament that surrounds the radial head, the accessory ulna collateral ligament and the posterolateral ligament that inserts along the margin of the greater sigmoid notch posteriorly.

- Why is the radial head at risk of non-union or avascular necrosis after fracture?

    The radial head is an intracapsular structure that receives a blood supply from a branch of the radial recurrent artery that travels up the neck of the radius from distal to proximal and is at risk of disruption by fracture or surgery.

References

1. Keats TE, Teeslink R, Diamond AE, Williams JH. Normal axial relationships of the major joints. Radiology. 1966;87(5):904–7.
2. Alcid JG, Ahmad CS, Lee TQ. Elbow anatomy and structural biomechanics. Clin Sports Med. 2004;23(4):503–17, vii
3. Morrey BF, Askew LJ, Chao EY. A biomechanical study of normal functional elbow motion. J Bone Joint Surg Am. 1981;63(6):872–7.
4. Johansson O. Capsular and ligament injuries of the elbow joint. A clinical and arthrographic study. Acta chirurgica Scandinavica Supplementum. 1962;287(Suppl):1–159.
5. O'Driscoll SW, Jaloszynski R, Morrey BF, An KN. Origin of the medial ulnar collateral ligament. J Hand Surg. 1992;17(1):164–8.
6. Cage DJ, Abrams RA, Callahan JJ, Botte MJ. Soft tissue attachments of the ulnar coronoid process. An anatomic study with radiographic correlation. Clin Orthop Relat Res. 1995;320:154–8.
7. Ochi N, Ogura T, Hashizume H, Shigeyama Y, Senda M, Inoue H. Anatomic relation between the medial collateral ligament of the elbow and the humero-ulnar joint axis. J Shoulder Elbow Surg. 1999;8(1):6–10. American Shoulder and Elbow Surgeons [et al].
8. Regan WD, Korinek SL, Morrey BF, An KN. Biomechanical study of ligaments around the elbow joint. Clin Orthop Relat Res. 1991;271:170–9.
9. Floris S, Olsen BS, Dalstra M, Sojbjerg JO, Sneppen O. The medial collateral ligament of the elbow joint: anatomy and kinematics. J Shoulder Elbow Surg. 1998;7(4):345–51. American Shoulder and Elbow Surgeons [et al].
10. Schwab GH, Bennett JB, Woods GW, Tullos HS. Biomechanics of elbow instability: the role of the medial collateral ligament. Clin Orthop Relat Res. 1980;146:42–52.
11. Morrey BF, An KN. Functional anatomy of the ligaments of the elbow. Clin Orthop Relat Res. 1985;201:84–90.
12. O'Driscoll SW, Bell DF, Morrey BF. Posterolateral rotatory instability of the elbow. J Bone Joint Surg. 1991;73(3):440–6. American volume.
13. de Seze MP, Rezzouk J, de Seze M, Uzel M, Lavignolle B, Midy D, et al. Does the motor branch of the long head of the triceps brachii arise from the radial nerve? An anatomic and electromyographic study. Surg Radiol Anat. 2004;26(6):459–61.
14. McCann PA, Smith GC, Clark D, Amirfeyz R. The tricipital aponeurosis – a reliable soft tissue landmark for humeral plating. Hand Surg. 2015;20(1):53–8. An international journal devoted to hand and upper limb surgery and related research : journal of the Asia-Pacific Federation of Societies for Surgery of the Hand.
15. Calfee RP, Wilson JM, Wong AH. Variations in the anatomic relations of the posterior interosseous nerve associated with proximal forearm trauma. J Bone Joint Surg. 2011;93(1):81–90.
16. Spinner M. The anterior interosseous-nerve syndrome, with special attention to its variations. J Bone Joint Surg. 1970;52(1):84–94. American volume.
17. Dellon AL, MacKinnon SE. Injury to the medial antebrachial cutaneous nerve during cubital tunnel surgery. J Hand Surg. 1985;10(1):33–6.
18. Yamaguchi K, Sweet FA, Bindra R, Morrey BF, Gelberman RH. The extraosseous and intraosseous arterial anatomy of the adult elbow. J Bone Joint Surg. 1997;79(11):1653–62. American volume.

Imaging of the Elbow

2

James R. A. Smith and Rouin Amirfeyz

Contents

Key Learning Points

1. Plain radiographs are the most common initial imaging modality for the elbow.
2. MRI is useful for examining soft tissue pathology but particular scans are required for individual pathology e.g. FABS views for distal biceps tendon pathology. Addition of contrast can enhance identification of pathology.
3. CT is used to examine bony pathology such as in acute fractures.
4. Ultrasound is examiner dependent but can be a useful tool for dynamic examination of the joint or to guide therapeutic injection.

J. R. A. Smith
Severn Deanery, Bristol, UK

R. Amirfeyz (✉)
Bristol Royal Infirmary, Bristol, UK
e-mail: rouin.amirfeyz@uhbristol.nhs.uk

© The Editor(s) (if applicable) and The Author(s), under exclusive license to Springer Nature Switzerland AG 2021
A. C. Watts et al. (eds.), *Sports Injuries of the Elbow*, https://doi.org/10.1007/978-3-030-52379-4_2

2.1   Introduction

Due to complexity of the anatomy and mechanics of the elbow, imaging plays an essential role in the examination of the injured joint. This review summarises the different modalities available to the treating physician, followed by a section outlining imaging for the most commonly encountered elbow disorders.

2.2   Imaging Modalities

2.2.1   Radiography

Plain radiographs are the first line of investigation, providing an overview of the osseous structures, the joint space and the soft tissues. A minimum of anteroposterior (AP) and lateral projections are necessary.

The AP view is taken with the elbow fully extended, and the forearm in full supination. It allows assessment of the medial and lateral epicondyles, radiocapitellar and trochlear joint surfaces (Fig. 2.1).

The lateral view is taken with the elbow flexed to 90°, with the forearm in neutral rotation. It allows good visualisation of the olecranon and coronoid processes. An appropriately taken lateral elbow radiograph demonstrates three concentric circles in various sizes. The smallest is the projection of the central part of the trochlea (groove), the middle is from the capitellum (projecting towards the radial head) and the largest corresponds to the medial ridge of the trochlea (mainly extending distally) (Fig. 2.2).

Oblique, radial head and axial views are now uncommonly performed due to the widespread availability of computer tomography scanning [1]. Joint effusions can be seen indirectly via displacement of the soft tissue shadows (Fig. 2.3), and elevation of the anterior or posterior fat pads on the lateral radiograph may indicate subtle intra-articular fluid from inflammation or occult fracture [2] (Fig. 2.4).

Periarticular densities are often visible on plain radiography, which is useful in diagnosing conditions such as crystal arthropathy, calcific tendonitis or hypertrophic ossification.

Fig. 2.1 Anteroposterior radiograph of the elbow

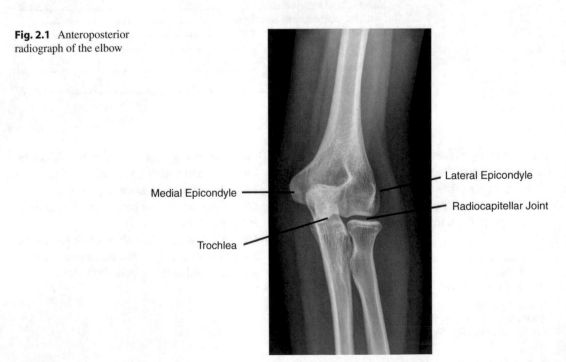

Medial Epicondyle

Trochlea

Lateral Epicondyle

Radiocapitellar Joint

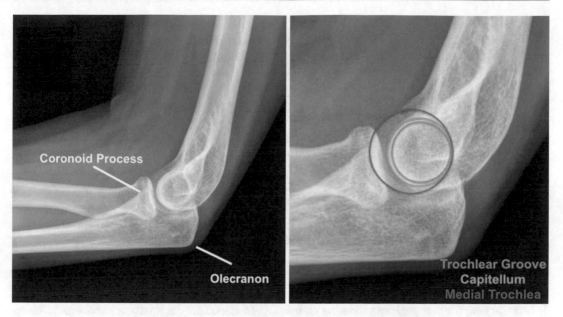

Fig. 2.2 Lateral radiograph of the elbow

Fig. 2.3 Anteroposterior radiograph demonstrating a joint effusion and radial head fracture

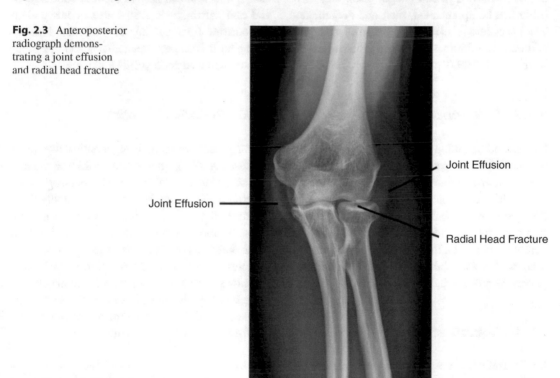

2.2.2 Fluoroscopy

Fluoroscopic assisted examination under anaesthetic is arguably the "gold-standard" method for assessment of subacute and chronic elbow instability as there is no muscle contraction or guarding to mask instability. This can be performed with patient supine, the shoulder flexed to 90° and the examiner standing at the head of the table supporting the affected arm. The C-arm

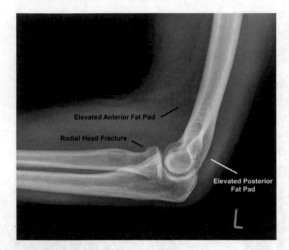

Fig. 2.4 'Raised fat pad' sign

is brought over the top of patient focusing on the elbow (usually a lateral image). This way instability can be appreciated, seen and documented. The procedure is usually scheduled as a day-case and once the findings discussed with the patient, further treatment is planned.

2.2.3 Ultrasonography

Ultrasound scanning (US) is non-invasive, well tolerated by the patient, dynamic and repeatable. Colour Doppler can be used to demonstrate blood flow changes that might indicate conditions such as tendinopathy, synovitis or bursitis. It is operator dependent, however, and it is difficult to derive much information from saved static images. US may be used to guide therapeutic injections around the elbow.

2.2.4 Computed Tomography (CT)

CT is useful for defining complex fracture patterns, occult fractures, osteochondral defects and articular pathology. When there is a need for an accurate understanding of the bony anatomy (such as planning for surgical treatment of heterotopic ossification, corrective osteotomy or arthroplasty in bone loss) CT scan is the imaging modality of choice. Combining with an intra-articular contrast injection can further define the anatomy in

the presence of a seemingly idiopathic restricted elbow motion, identifying synovial thickening and loose bodies [3].

2.2.5 Magnetic Resonance Imaging (MRI)

MRI allows high-resolution imaging of ligaments, tendons, neurovascular structures, articular cartilage and subchondral bone [4], and is, therefore, well-suited to the investigation of elbow pathology. It is also very valuable in cases of occult fractures and "bone bruises" not identifiable with radiograph or CT scan. It is preferable to USS when multiple anatomical structures need imaging simultaneously.

Intraarticular contrast (commonly gadolinium-based) injection can help to identify subtle synovial and cartilage defects, loose bodies and to demonstrate ligament injuries, whereas intravenous gadolinium provides enhancement of other lesions such as osteomyelitis and neoplasia.

2.2.6 Bone Scintigraphy

A 'bone scan' works by using a radioactive tracer (technetium 99m), attached to methylene diphosphonate, which is taken up by osteoblasts and, therefore, acts a marker of bone activity. The gamma radiation emitted is processed by a gamma camera to form an image. Bone scanning is useful in the diagnosis of neoplasia, osteomyelitis, stress fractures, avascular necrosis, arthritis, and prosthetic loosening when used in conjunction with primary imaging. However, this modality is used less frequently as CT & MRI are more readily available and the images obtained are more detailed.

2.3 Common Elbow Conditions

2.3.1 Acute Trauma

The majority of adult elbow fractures can be diagnosed on plain radiographs, appearing as a lucency on either the AP or lateral radiograph (Fig. 2.5).

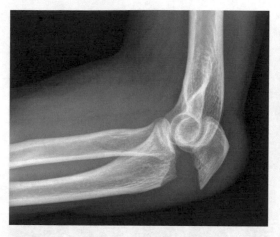

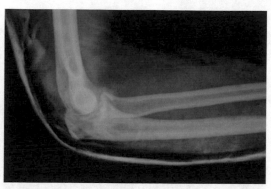

Fig. 2.6 Lateral radiograph demonstrating a coronoid fracture

Fig. 2.5 Lateral radiograph demonstrating an olecranon fracture

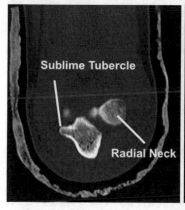

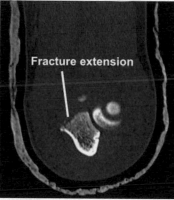

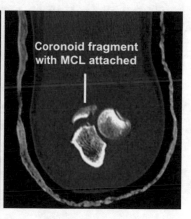

Fig. 2.7 Axial view of coronoid, demonstrating a fracture of the anteromedial facet. This is often associated with a lateral ligament avulsion, and therefore osseoligamentous instability

Minimally displaced fractures may present as a raised fat pad sign, and the majority of these in adults will represent radial head fractures [5].

CT scanning is best used to define fracture comminution and configuration [6]. It is particularly useful when assessing coronoid fractures (Fig. 2.6) to delineate the position of the fracture line in relation to the sublime tubercle (insertion of the anterior bundle of MCL), therefore, determining valgus stability of the elbow (Fig. 2.7). CT is also very valuable in surgical planning for complex cases such as comminuted proximal ulna fracture with or without proximal radioulnar joint dislocation.

MRI is valuable in detecting occult fractures, osteochondral defects, bone bruising and collateral ligament tears [7].

2.3.2 Ligamentous Instability

Medial collateral ligamentous insufficiency can be due to an acute valgus injury, or from repetitive strain as seen in throwing athletes. Plain radiographs are of limited value, though will demonstrate bony avulsions or heterotopic ossification in chronic cases. Small osteophyte formation on the medial tip of the olecranon seen on an AP view could point towards the diagnosis of valgus extension overload. Valgus stress views are of some value, but MCL laxity has been demonstrated to be a normal finding in asymptomatic throwing athletes [8]. The best way to assess and compare to the unaffected side is fluoroscopic assisted examination under anaesthetic.

Ultrasound can identify tears of the MCL, and dynamic scanning can be performed with the elbow under valgus stress to confirm or exclude complete tears [9]. Full thickness tears appear as a discontinuity of the ligament with intervening fluid.

Magnetic resonance arthrogram is the investigation of choice, and can demonstrate subtle partial tears. It can also identify marrow oedema in chronic stress when no rupture is visible. Coincidental injuries of the elbow are identifiable on the scan.

Lateral collateral ligament injuries can result in posterolateral rotatory instability [10]. Imaging principles are similar to that of the MCL with the majority of injuries diagnosed on MRI. Fluoroscopic-assisted examination under anaesthetic can help to demonstrate dynamic instability in conjunction with stress tests, such as the pivot shift and varus/valgus stress tests.

2.3.3 Musculotendinous Pathology

The distal biceps tendon is the most commonly injured tendon in the elbow, and ultrasonography is a good first-line investigation in the presence of inconclusive clinical signs [11]. Complete tears will show hypoechoic or anechoic fibre disruption, with or without tendon retraction. Partial tears appear as thickening of the tendon close to its insertion [11].

MRI is reliable in demonstrating distal biceps tendon complete rupture, partial rupture or tendinosis (Fig. 2.8). Although diagnosis of a complete rupture is clinical other aforementioned pathologies commonly require an MRI scan. The optimal position for scanning is Flexion of elbow, Abduction of shoulder and Supination of the forearm (so called FABS view) [12].

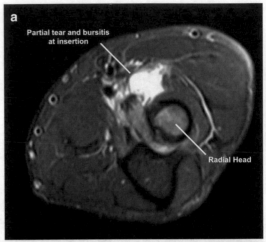

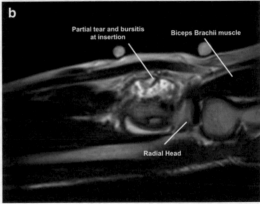

Fig. 2.8 (**a**) Partial tear and bursitis of distal biceps tendon—axial STIR sequence. (**b**) Partial tear and bursitis of distal biceps tendon—sagittal T2 sequence

Lateral and medial epicondylitis (so called tennis and golfer's elbow, respectively) are common elbow conditions potentially resulting from overuse. The pathology includes tendinosis, degeneration and tearing within the respective common extensor and flexor tendon origins. One should bear in mind that these conditions are generally diagnosed on clinical grounds and imaging modalities are to exclude the possibility of other pathologies if presenting symptoms are not typical. Plain radiographs are indicated in adolescents, the elderly, those with a history of trauma to the elbow and those with mechanical symptoms to exclude alternative pathology. Some practicing surgeons routinely radiograph elbows prior to operation to ensure no sinister pathology is missed.

Ultrasound demonstrates thickening, hypoechogenicity and hyperaemia on colour Doppler. USS has been shown to be as specific but not as sensitive as MRI [13] for diagnosing epicondylitis. MRI has the added benefit in evaluating any associated osseous oedema. Muscle strains are best seen on T2 weighted MRI imaging at the myotendinous junction.

2.3.4 Soft Tissue Masses and Swellings

Soft tissue swellings are common around the elbow, and the majority are located superficially. Ultrasonography is, therefore, a good initial modality to differentiate cystic and solid lesions, and can determine vascularity with the use of Doppler. Further differentiation from the surrounding tissues can be determined using MRI scanning.

Cystic lesions (ganglia, lipoma, haematoma, bursae) will appear hypo or anechoic on USS, and signal intense on fluid sensitive MRI sequences.

2.3.5 Olecranon and Bicipital Bursitis

USS can be used to confirm a fluid collection within the olecranon bursa. Due to its deeper location, the bicipitoradial bursa is best imaged using fluid sensitive MRI sequences.

The appearance of an infected bursa on MRI is not easily discernible, however, a lack of enhancement following intravenous gadolinium contrast injection usually excludes infection [14].

2.3.6 Entrapment Neuropathies

Imaging of suspected nerve entrapment allows the causative lesion to be identified, the integrity of the nerve to be assessed, and the secondary effects of the entrapment delineated.

Ulnar nerve entrapment in the cubital tunnel is the most common neuropathy around the elbow. USS will show nerve thickening proximal to any

compressive structure, and can be used dynamically to assess dislocation or subluxation of the nerve with elbow movement. On MRI, the nerve appears enlarged on all sequences, with high signal on T2 weighted images. Muscle denervation of compression neuropathy is also demonstrated on MRI as denervation oedema, muscle atrophy, myositis or fatty infiltration [15].

The median nerve can be compressed proximal to the elbow by a bony spur in the region of the ligament of Struthers, and stenosis of the brachial artery often occurs simultaneously. Plain radiographs will demonstrate the supracondylar spur, and both USS and MRI will show nerve thickening. USS Doppler and MR angiography may show associated artery stenosis. Compression of the median nerve may also occur as it passes between the two heads of pronator teres, causing pronator syndrome. MRI may show denervation atrophy/myositis, and can be used to differentiate between entrapment of the anterior interosseous nerve and median nerve proper, based upon the muscle group involved [15].

Radial nerve entrapment occurs at the arcade of Frohse, or as it passes through the supinator muscle. It is best imaged using MRI, where denervation myositis or fatty infiltration of the supinator and forearm extensor muscles is seen [16].

2.4 Conclusion

Multiple imaging modalities are available to aid in the diagnosis and management of elbow pathology. Each has particular strengths and limitations. Where there is uncertainty surrounding the best imaging tool to use for a specific problem it is recommended to consult with a specialist musculoskeletal radiologist.

Q&A
What imaging should you request to investigate a suspected partial tear of the distal biceps tendon?
The best imaging modality is plain magnetic resonance imaging, particularly with flexion abduction supination (FABS) views with a specific coil under the elbow. This allows visualisation of the whole tendon to the insertion in a

single slice and is more sensitive for detecting partial tears.

How can CT help in the management of acute elbow fractures?

CT can be used to understand fracture patterns around the elbow. CT will frequently show more extensive fragmentation than can be appreciated on plain radiographs, or reveal unseen additional injuries. It is particularly helpful in understanding elbow fracture dislocation injuries and distal humerus fractures. CT is often used by surgeons to plan fracture fixation.

When is ultrasound most useful in imaging of elbow pathology?

Ultrasound can be used to provide a dynamic assessment of elbow pathology and in combination with Doppler imaging, can show blood flow changes such as in tendinopathy or synovitis. US can also be used to guide injections for treatment of elbow pathology.

You have an athelete in whom you suspect a chronic lateral ligament injury. What imaging would you request to investigate further?

Chronic instability can be demonstrated in a number of ways. Fluoroscopy of the elbow can be used with stress views to demonstrate joint gapping or subluxation and permits a dynamic assessment of the elbow but may not be tolerated well in the awake patient. Ultrasound can show joint ligament discontinuity and joint gapping on stress views but is operator dependent. MR arthrography will demonstrate ligament and tendon avulsion injuries and can also show joint subluxation and bony injury. It has the advantage that it can be "read" remotely from saved images. CT arthrogram may be helpful for appreciation of combined chronic osseos and ligamentous instability.

References

1. Miller TT. Imaging of elbow disorders. Orthoped Clin N Am. 1999;30(1):21–36.
2. Goswami GK. The fat pad sign. Radiology. 2002;222(2):419–20.
3. Singson RD, Feldman F, Rosenberg ZS. Elbow joint: assessment with double-contrast CT arthrography. Radiology. 1986;160(1):167–73.
4. Yoshioka H, Ueno T, Tanaka T, Kujiraoka Y, Shindo M, Takahashi N, et al. High-resolution MR imaging of the elbow using a microscopy surface coil and a clinical 1.5 T MR machine: preliminary results. Skelet Radiol. 2004;33(5):265–71.
5. O'Dwyer H, O'Sullivan P, Fitzgerald D, Lee MJ, McGrath F, Logan PM. The fat pad sign following elbow trauma in adults: its usefulness and reliability in suspecting occult fracture. J Comput Assist Tomogr. 2004;28(4):562–5.
6. Haapamaki VV, Kiuru MJ, Koskinen SK. Multidetector computed tomography diagnosis of adult elbow fractures. Acta Radiol. 2004;45(1):65–70.
7. Brunton LM, Anderson MW, Pannunzio ME, Khanna AJ, Chhabra AB. Magnetic resonance imaging of the elbow: update on current techniques and indications. J Hand Surg. 2006;31(6):1001–11.
8. Singh H, Osbahr DC, Wickham MQ, Kirkendall DT, Speer KP. Valgus laxity of the ulnar collateral ligament of the elbow in collegiate athletes. Am J Sports Med. 2001;29(5):558–61.
9. De Smet AA, Winter TC, Best TM, Bernhardt DT. Dynamic sonography with valgus stress to assess elbow ulnar collateral ligament injury in baseball pitchers. Skelet Radiol. 2002;31(11):671–6.
10. O'Driscoll SW, Bell DF, Morrey BF. Posterolateral rotatory instability of the elbow. J Bone Joint Surg. 1991;73(3):440–6. American volume.
11. Miller TT, Adler RS. Sonography of tears of the distal biceps tendon. AJR Am J Roentgenol. 2000;175(4):1081–6.
12. Giuffre BM, Moss MJ. Optimal positioning for MRI of the distal biceps brachii tendon: flexed abducted supinated view. AJR Am J Roentgenol. 2004;182(4):944–6.
13. Miller TT, Shapiro MA, Schultz E, Kalish PE. Comparison of sonography and MRI for diagnosing epicondylitis. J Clin Ultrasound. 2002;30(4):193–202.
14. Floemer F, Morrison WB, Bongartz G, Ledermann HP. MRI characteristics of olecranon bursitis. AJR Am J Roentgenol. 2004;183(1):29–34.
15. Kim S, Choi JY, Huh YM, Song HT, Lee SA, Kim SM, et al. Role of magnetic resonance imaging in entrapment and compressive neuropathy – what, where, and how to see the peripheral nerves on the musculoskeletal magnetic resonance image: Part 1. Overview and lower extremity. Eur Radiol. 2007;17(1):139–49.
16. Ferdinand BD, Rosenberg ZS, Schweitzer ME, Stuchin SA, Jazrawi LM, Lenzo SR, et al. MR imaging features of radial tunnel syndrome: initial experience. Radiology. 2006;240(1):161–8.

Biomechanics of the Elbow Joint

3

Jeppe Vejlgaard Rasmussen
and Bo Sanderhoff Olsen

Contents

3.1 Introduction

The elbow joint allows positioning of the hand inside a sphere around the body, created by the shoulder movement and with the length of the arm as the radius. It is the second link, in a chain of joint levers, that begins at the shoulder and ends at the fingers. Therefore, elbow joint pathology may severely affect the function of the upper extremity, and more specifically, the ability of the individual to position and fixate the hand, necessary for the use of the hand in work and leisure activities [1–3] (Fig. 3.1).

The anatomy is relatively complex. The joint consists of articulations between the humerus, ulna and radius with three different articulations mediating two directions of movement, namely a

J. V. Rasmussen · B. S. Olsen (✉)
Section for surgery of the Shoulder and the Elbow,
Orthopedic Department T, Copenhagen University
Hospital, Herlev/Gentofte Hospital,
Hellerup, Denmark
e-mail: Jeppe.Vejlgaard.Rasmussen@regionh.dk;
Bo.Sanderhoff.Olsen@regionh.dk

A. C. Watts et al. (eds.), *Sports Injuries of the Elbow*, https://doi.org/10.1007/978-3-030-52379-4_3

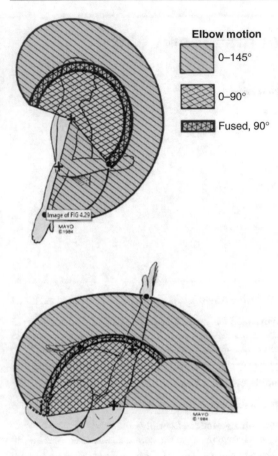

Elbow motion

- ▨ 0–145°
- ▩ 0–90°
- ▦ Fused, 90°

Fig. 3.1 The shoulder motion allows positioning of the hand on a sphere around the body, with the arm-length as the diameter. The elbow motion allows positioning of the hand inside this sphere (Morrey's the Elbow and its Disorders 5th edition 2017)

so called hinge joint flexion and extension axis and a pivoting or rotating motion around the fore-arm axis. The elbow hinge joint motion is mediated by the ulnohumeral and the radiohumeral joints. The forearm pivoting or rotating motion is mediated by the proximal radioulnar and the radiohumeral joints. Therefore, the elbow joint is described as a composite trocho-gynglymoid joint [2, 3].

In the present text we will focus on the biomechanics and kinematics of the elbow joint, that allows its delicate function, with special focus on the clinical important entities of the joint mechanism.

3.2 Ranges of Motion and Carrying Angle

The elbow joint motion is described around different axes allowing functional elbow flexion-extension and forearm rotation defined as pronation-supination respectively [4].

Normally, the motion in flexion and extension is defined as full extension 0° and flexion to the soft tissues normally described at 145°. Pronation and supination are normally described in 90° elbow flexion, since this stabilises humeral rotation. At this position pronation is usually 80° and supination approximately 90° [5]. Active motion is usually less than passive motion. With age, motion decreases and gender has an influence; females are more prone to hyperextension than males [4, 5].

In 1981, Morrey et al. [6] examined the motion necessary for performing an array of everyday activities. These authors defined an elbow flexion axis between 30° and 130° and a forearm rotation axis of 50° supination to 50° pronation as necessary for leading a normal life. Nowadays, this motion axis might be insufficient for most people and especially for athletes (Fig. 3.2).

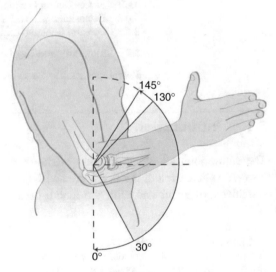

Fig. 3.2 This is a graphic presentation of the motion of the elbow joint with a presentation of the range of motion defined by Morrey et al. as the minimum required motion necessary for performing simple every day activities (Morrey's the Elbow and its Disorders 5th edition 2017)

The carrying angle is defined as the lateral deviation of the forearm relative to the upper arm seen in full elbow extension. The angle is diminished with flexion and in full flexion the forearm covers the upper arm. This is due to the fact that the hinge axis is abducted one-half of the carrying angle, relative to the sagittal plane of the humerus, as described by Amis et al. [5, 7]. The carrying angle is more pronounced in females were it averages up to 14°; less in males. Furthermore, it increases through puberty (Amis [5]) (Fig. 3.3).

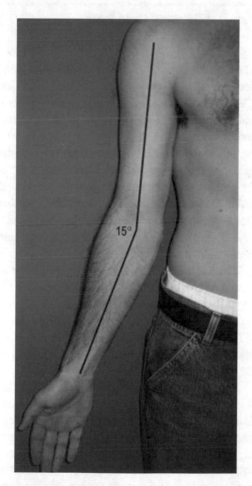

Fig. 3.3 The carrying angle is the lateral deviation of the forearm relative to the upper arm, seen in extension but disappears in full flexion (Operative Elbow Surgery 1st edition, 2012)

3.3 Muscles Inducing Motion

The muscles of the elbow are traditionally described according to the primary motion they induce. The biceps brachii, the brachialis, and the brachioradialis muscles induce flexion, the triceps brachii muscle extension, and the supinator and the pronator teres muscles forearm rotation. The other muscles in the elbow region provides various but limited contribution to the active elbow motion and will not be further discussed.

3.3.1 Flexor Muscles

The larger superficial head of the brachialis muscle originates from a large area on the anterolateral part of the middle-third of the humerus and inserts on the coronoid process just distal from the articular margin. The smaller deep head originates more distally than the superficial head. Some of the fibres end as a sagittal oriented aponeurosis inserting on the ulna. Others fibres insert on the anterior joint capsule and may prevent impingement during flexion [8]. The brachialis muscle has the largest cross-sectional area of the flexors but the force induced by the muscle is impaired by the short distance from the insertion to the axis of rotation [9] (Fig. 3.4).

The other major flexor is the biceps brachii muscle. It has a short and a long head originating from the coracoid process and the superior aspect of the glenoid, respectively. The anteromedial part of the muscle and the fasciae continue as the bicipital aponeurosis and inserts to the deep muscle fasciae of the forearm, whereas the biceps tendon inserts to the posterior aspect of the radial tuberosity. The biomechanics are intermediate compared to that of the brachialis and the brachioradialis muscles. The biceps brachii is not only a flexor but also a strong supinator [10].

The brachioradialis muscle has a lengthy origin on the distal lateral aspect of the humerus and inserts into the base of the radial styloid. The cross-sectional area of the muscle is small compared with that of the brachialis and the biceps brachii muscles, but the longer distance from the

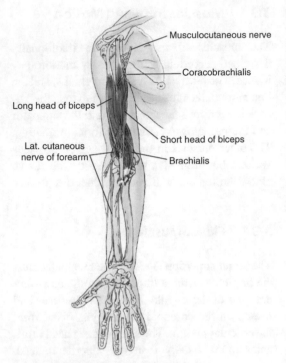

Musculocutaneous nerve

Coracobrachialis

Long head of biceps

Short head of biceps

Lat. cutaneous
nerve of forearm

Brachialis

Fig. 3.4 The short distance from the insertion of the brachialis and the biceps brachii muscles to the axis of rotation is associated with biomechanical disadvantages (Morrey's the Elbow and its Disorders 5th edition 2017)

insertion to the axis of rotation gives biomechanical advantages [9] (Fig. 3.4).

3.3.2 Extensor Muscles

The triceps brachii is a large extensor muscle with the largest cross-sectional area of the elbow muscles. It has three heads: the long head originates from the infraglenoid tuberosity; the lateral head from the proximal posterolateral part of the humerus; and the medial head from the distal posteromedial aspect of the humerus, which is muscular almost to its insertion. Distally the muscle merges into one tendon that mainly inserts around the olecranon process [11].

3.3.3 Forearm Rotation

The supinator is a flat rhomboid muscle with three origins proximal or distal to the elbow joint.

It is running obliquely from the anterior part of the lateral epicondyle, the lateral collateral ligament and the proximal part on the crest of ulna to the diffuse insertion on a larger part of the proximal radius. The muscle is characterised by the absence of tendinous tissue [12].

The pronator teres muscle origins from the anterior aspect of the medial epicondyle and from the coronoid process. It inserts into the junction between the proximal and the middle-third of the radius. It obviously contributes to pronation of the forearm, but it is also considered as a weak flexor muscle [13, 14].

3.4 Kinematics of Bony Stabilisers

The humeroulnar joint has a high congruency between the deep humeral trochlea and the greater sigmoid notch of the ulna, inducing bony stability, enhanced by the strong side ligaments and the muscle forces acting over the joint. The top of the radial head, with its concavity, and the spherical capitellum that articulates with concavity compression increases the bony constraint and is further constrained by the annular ligament that surrounds the radial head [15].

Below we will focus on different bony and ligamentous constraints.

The **radial head** is a secondary stabiliser to forced valgus, acting as a buttress against the capitellum [16]. More studies describe the influence of the radial head in elbow joint stability [17–19]. Isolated resection of the radial head gives minor laxity to forced varus and forced external rotation (Fig. 3.5).

The stabilising effect may be caused partly by tensioning of the Lateral Collateral Ligament Complex (LCLC) [17]. Combined radial head resection and dissection of the Medial Collateral Ligament (MCL) induces grave laxity to forced valgus and forced internal rotation [18]. Radial head resection and injury to the Radial Collateral Ligament (RCL) increases the laxity seen after isolated RCL incision in forced varus and external rotation. No changes in laxity to forced valgus and internal rotation are observed in this situation [19].

Fig. 3.5 Isolated radial resection gives minor rotatory laxity to forced external rotation [17]

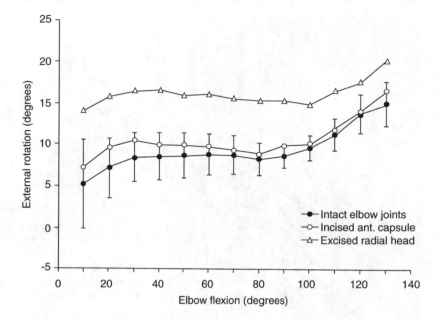

More than 2/3 of the radial head has to be intact in order to preserve joint stability in forced valgus and varus [20].

Differences in radiohumeral stability to forced translation, related to the radial position on the capitellum, indicates an inherent stability in the radiohumeral joint related to differences in wall height around the radial head; so called concavity compression [21].

This further emphasises that the radio-capitellar articulation induces joint stability as a unit. Therefore, a capitellum fracture has the same potential for causing elbow-instability as reported for the radial head, except for the stabilising effect induced by the radial head through tensioning of the LCLC. A loaded model on elbow joint dislocation, showed the radial head to possess a minor, though primary, constraint against elbow joint dislocation [22].

The radial head, along with the coronoid process, induces axial stability to the elbow [23]. A combination of elbow dislocation and fracture of both structures was defined as the terrible triad by Hotchkiss [24], due to the severe elbow instability it might cause. At least one of the two is needed in order to preserve clinical joint stability [22, 23].

The coronoid process is an important elbow joint stabiliser [22–27]. Fractures of the coronoid

process are often associated with dislocation of the elbow, and the coronoid fracture might indicate a severely unstable situation [23, 24]. Fractures can be defined according to their extension into the coronoid process [28, 29].

Research has shown that isolated coronoid process resection Regan stage II (50%) induces significant laxity to "dislocation", decreasing the joint constraint up to 28% [22]. Another study emphasised that, in ligamentous and radial-head deficient elbows, at least 50% of the process was needed in order to prevent posterior elbow translation. In coronoid process injury, joints are more stable in flexion [26]. Increasing coronoid process resection gives increasing alterations in joint kinematics. Type I injury is reported to produce only minor changes in joint constraint, type II injury or more, significantly affects the valgus-varus constraint. Laxity induced by coronoid resection is less in forearm supination than in pronation [25]. However, the combination of anteromedial coronoid fractures and LCL insufficiency was shown to induce posteromedial elbow joint instability [27]. This emphasised the need for surgical fixation of anteromedial facet fractures and LCL reinsertion in this clinical situation [27, 30] (Fig. 3.6).

Transection of the proximal ulna/olecranon was observed to increase laxity of the elbow joint

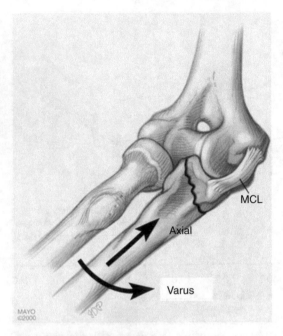

Fig. 3.6 The cause for posteromedial elbow instability in anteromedial coronoid process fractures [30]

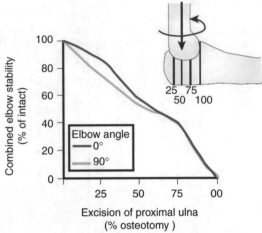

Fig. 3.7 Staged olecranon process resection gives linear decrease in combined elbow joint instability (Morrey's the Elbow and its Disorders 5th edition, 2017)

to valgus and varus stress. The instability was increased in a linear way following staged olecranon resections. It was observed though, that the proximal part primarily resists valgus loads and the inferior part primarily resists varus loads. Rotatory loads where not evaluated. Therefore, the most proximal part of the olecranon process could be removed in case of comminuted fracture, without inducing clinical significant joint instability [31] (Fig. 3.7).

Posteromedial olecranon resection gave an increased valgus laxity following minor olecranon resections in a setting with intact MCL [32]. This led these authors to recommend caution in surgical resection of the proximal olecranon especially among throwing athletes, where insufficiency of the MCL could be suspected [32].

3.5 Kinematics of Soft Tissue Stabilisers

The soft tissue stabilisers constitute the muscles described above and the joint capsule, with ligamentous reinforcements medially and laterally,

described as the medial and lateral collateral ligament complexes respectively.

We know that several large muscles cross the elbow joint, but their stabilising effect on the joint are difficult to document. Loading of experimental elbow models reduces the laxity induced to the elbow joint specimens by osteoligamentous divisions, but the passive stabilising effect of the muscular tendons were only minor [33, 34]. Clinically, a muscular hypotonia following a dislocation was observed, and it was speculated that this might increase the immediate joint instability [19]. Furthermore, it is well known that the flexor and extensor origins might be avulsed or ruptured along with the ligaments in the clinical situation with an elbow dislocation [35].

The posterior capsule is usually relatively thin, compared with the thicker anterior capsule. Both are reported to be torn following elbow joint dislocation [35]. Originally, the anterior capsule was reported to be an important stabiliser in elbow joint extension [36]. Other studies documented that with preserved ligaments, no specific laxity was induced after capsular transection other than what was caused by the inherent negative intraarticular pressure, except in full elbow joint extension [17, 37]. In this extended position the stabilising influence of the capsule to forced external rotation actually exceeded that of the LCL [38]. O'Driscoll et al. [39] showed that capsular resection associated with LCL injury was necessary to bring the elbow joint into the so-called "perched position", indicating some kind of secondary stabilising effect of the capsular tissue does exist.

Following a dislocation of the elbow joint, bilateral ligament injury has been documented [35]. Although the usual reported cause for insufficiency of the MCL is valgus stress among throwing athletes, the LCL injury often relates to elbow trauma with dislocation [15]. The circle concept is an experimental model that describes the different stages in an elbow joint dislocation related to ligamentous injury [39].

The MCL is divided into the anterior- and the posterior-bundle (AB and PB, respectively) and the transverse ligament. The AB extends from the medial epicondyle and inserts on the medial side of the coronoid process, is described as the strongest part with a mean load to failure of 260 N [40]. Different bands in the anterior bundle are described [41]. This ligament is perceived as a continuum of fibres that induces constraint with increasing joint flexion from anterior to posterior [40, 41, 42, 43] (Fig. 3.8).

The PB is a fan-shaped thickening of the capsule somewhat thinner than the AB, it extends from the medial epicondyle and inserts on the medial side of the olecranon [41, 43].

The transverse ligament extends from the medial tip of the olecranon to the medial side of the processus coronoideus. The structure is difficult to see and no stability induced to the elbow is detected [43].

There are more reports on the stability induced to the elbow by the MCL [16 18, 36, 38–43]. Transection of the AB induced significant elbow joint laxity to forced valgus and internal rotation, with a maximal laxity at 70° elbow flexion. The anterior part of the AB stabilises in extension, whereas the most posterior fibres stabilise the elbow in flexion. PB transection alone gave no joint laxity, but in combination with AB it increased the observed laxity, with a maximum laxity at 90° elbow flexion [41]. In another study, surgical AB reconstruction normalised joint stability in total MCL transection [18]. Forearm supination tends to stabilise a MCL deficient elbow joint [44]. Overall, these findings were confirmed in other experimental studies [16, 18, 40, 42, 43] (Fig. 3.8).

The LCLC is divided into the annular ligament and the lateral collateral ligament (LCL) made from the radial collateral ligament (RCL) that extends down from the undersurface of the lateral epicondyle and inserts into the annular ligament (AL), and more posteriorly are fibres that insert distal to the AL on the proximal supinator crest of the ulna—the lateral ulnar collateral ligament (LUCL) [45–47]. Separation of the different bands is difficult [48]. The AL surrounds the radial head and inserts on the anterior and posterior margins of the lesser sigmoid notch [43, 45–47].

Fig. 3.8 Describes the valgus forced laxity introduced to the elbow by serial sectioning of the different bands in the medial ligament complex [41]. The anterior bundle describes the AMCL, the anterior band is the anterior band of the AMCL, and the posterior band is the posterior band in the AMCL. The posterior bundle describes the PMCL

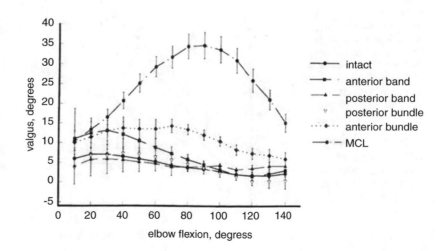

Recent studies showed that separate sectioning of the AL and the LUCL gave insignificant laxity to the elbow, whereas isolated RCL dissection gave major significant laxity to forced varus and external rotation, the laxity was largest at 100° of elbow joint flexion. Further dissection of the LUCL and AL increased the laxity significantly [46, 47]. Reconstruction of the LUCL, between the humeral epicondyle and the ulna, was shown to normalise elbow constraint in the LCLC deficient elbow joint specimens [47, 48]. Furthermore, recent research observed that forearm pronation and muscle loading tends to stabilise the LCLC deficient elbow [33, 38]. The results on elbow joint laxity following LCLC injury were confirmed by other experimental studies [19, 38, 49, 50] (Fig. 3.9).

Intensive studies on posterolateral elbow instability as described by O'Driscoll et al. [39, 45, 51] showed that isolated dissection of the LUCL gave no laxity to the Pivot Shift Stress Test (PST) [48, 51]. Another experimental study confirmed that only complete LCL transection introduced so-called pathological external forearm rotation, necessary for an elbow joint dislocation to occur [38]. Furthermore, LCL reconstruction was observed to stabilise the joint to PST [48]. Other experimental studies made the same observations [49, 50].

3.6 Forces Around the Elbow During Motion, Loading and Transmission Along the Forearm

The elbow joint is often falsely referred to as non-weight-bearing, but the load applied to the elbow joints can be heavy, as the forces induced by the elbow muscles balance the loading at the forearm and hand. The reasons for this are related to biomechanical disadvantages: the large distance from the axis of rotation to an external load in the hand; the short distance from the axis of rotation to the insertion of the tendons of the elbow muscles; and finally, in order to stabilise the joint during motion, the force induced is counteracted by antagonistic muscles.

3.6.1 Forces During Flexion

The required elbow forces in 90° of flexion are much higher than the external load applied to the hand. The reason for this is the large distance from the axis of rotation to an external load in the hand, the short distance from the axis of rotation to the insertion of the brachialis and biceps brachii muscles and the triceps muscle acting as an

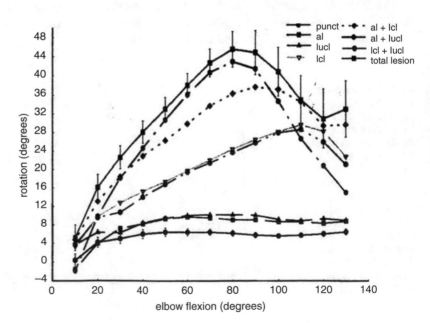

Fig. 3.9 Describes the external rotatory loaded laxity introduced to the elbow by serial sectioning of the different bands in the lateral ligament complex [47]. Punct.: describes the joint after puncture of the negative intraarticular pressure but with preservation of the joint capsule, AL: annular ligament, LUCL: lateral ulnar collateral ligament, LCL: lateral collateral ligament, Total lesion: LCLC incision

antagonist [52]. Since the brachialis muscle inserts on ulna and the biceps brachii, the brachioradialis and the pronator teres muscles on radius both the radiohumeral joint and the ulnohumeral joint can be loaded heavily during flexion [53] (Fig. 3.10).

The contribution of the individual muscles can be estimated as changes in electrical activity with use of electromyographic (EMG) examinations. It has been suggested that the individual flexor muscles are influenced by forearm rotation. With the elbow at 90° of flexion and with the forearm in neutral position the activity of the individual muscles is similar; however, with the forearm in maximum pronation the activity of the biceps brachii muscle is limited [54]. This is most likely related to the secondary role of the muscle as a supinator. In contrast, the activity of the brachioradialis muscle is increased in this position [54, 55]. The activity of the brachialis muscle seems to be independent of rotation of the forearm [10, 54]. Since the biceps brachii muscle act as a supinator too, it is worth noting that the pronator teres muscle has a high activity during elbow flexion insuring rotational equilibrium.

3.6.2 Extension

The medial head of the triceps brachii is the principle extensor. The lateral and the long head contribute as the load increases [11, 56, 57]. Because of the large cross sectional area of the muscle and biomechanical disadvantages, the load applied on the ulnohumeral joint is significantly and approximately 20 times larger than the external load applied to the hand [53]. The biceps brachii muscle and the flexor muscles act as antagonist during extension, so the required force from the triceps muscle is even higher [52].

3.6.3 Forearm Rotation

The forces during supination are induced by the biceps brachii muscle and, to a lesser extent, by the supinator muscle; whereas the pronation is induced by the pronator teres muscle, supported by the pronator quadratus muscle on the distal part of the forearm [58]. Except for the biceps brachii muscle the forearm rotation muscles mainly act transversely between radius and ulna. Thus, the forces on the radiohumeral and the

Fig. 3.10 The forces of the elbow flexor muscles has to balance the weight of the forearm and the load applied to the hand. Because of the large distance from the axis of rotation to the load applied to the hand, the weight of the forearm, and the short distance from the insertion of the flexor muscles to the axis of rotation, the load applied to the elbow joint can be heavy (Operative Elbow Surgery 1st edition, 2012)

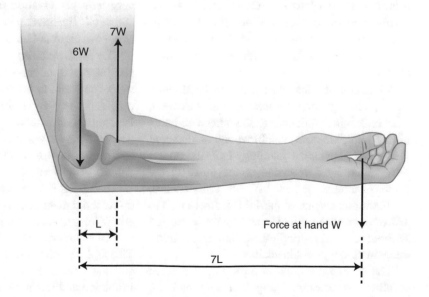

ulnohumeral joint during rotation of the forearm are limited [5]. The forearm rotation muscles are relatively small and the forces on the proximal and the distal radioulnar joint are smaller than the axial joint loads during flexion and extension [5].

3.7   Summary and Key Learning Points

The elbow is a very constrained joint due to the osseous structures, muscle forces acting across the joint, and capsuloligamentous structures. The joint motion is divided in hinge motion of flexion and extension and forearm rotation in pronation and supination.

The joint motion is normally 0–140° in flexion and extension and 80–90° in pronation and supination. Females and young individuals are more mobile. The carrying angle describes the lateral angle of the extended elbow and is caused by the abducted hinge axis of the joint.

The muscles of the elbow are traditionally described according to the primary motion they induce. The biceps brachii, the brachialis, and the brachioradialis muscles induce flexion; the triceps brachii muscle extension, and the supinator and the pronator teres muscles induce forearm rotation. Some of these muscles are, however, involved in more than one motion. The biceps brachii muscle is a strong supinator and the pronator teres muscle is considered a weak flexor muscle.

Kinematic studies indicate that isolated radial head pathology may be treated with resection, with only minor influence to the otherwise intact elbow joint; whereas, combinations of ligament injury and radial head pathology indicate caution with radial head resection, since grave elbow joint instability might be the consequence. Furthermore, displaced partial fractures of up to 1/3 of the radial head diameter might be treated without surgical reinsertion, without major influence on elbow joint kinematics.

The coronoid process is a primary constraint to elbow dislocation, acting as a bony buttress. Minor fractures of the coronoid process may be clinically insignificant, whereas, coronoid deficiency of >50% seriously affects the joint constraint. The joint laxity induced by resection seems to diminish with forearm supination. The observed joint laxity is present in the entire flexion axis, though the coronoid process may contribute more to elbow stability in extension than in flexion. Anteromedial facet fractures of the coronoid may indicate MCL insufficiency and calls for clinical attention.

The top of the olecranon induces valgus constraint and the inferior olecranon varus constraint to the elbow joint. With partial resection of the olecranon the laxity of the elbow is increased in a linear way. In throwing athletes with posterior elbow pain, caution with posteromedial olecranon resections is indicated.

The muscles probably act for stability through muscle-forces across the joint, compressing the congruent joint surfaces together. In this way, an early motion regimen with muscle activation might increase joint stability, following an acute simple elbow joint dislocation.

The anterior capsule does induce stability to the elbow joint in full extension, whereas in all other degrees of elbow joint position it acts along with the posterior capsule only as a secondary elbow joint stabiliser. Therefore, in elbow surgery with preservation or reconstruction of the collateral ligaments, surgical capsular reconstruction might not be necessary.

The MCL stabilises the elbow joint to valgus and internal rotatory stress. The AB is the primary constraint to both valgus and internal rotation and the PB is the secondary constraint. Isolated reconstruction of the AB in the MCL deficient elbow tends to normalise elbow constraint. Supination tends to stabilise the MCL deficient elbow joint.

The LCLC is a continuum of fibres more than discreet ligament bands. The LCLC stabilises the elbow joint to forced varus and external rotation, as well as to posterolateral elbow joint instability. The LCL is the primary constraint and the AL and the LUCL are only secondary constraints. Pronation and loading tends to stabilise the LCL deficient elbow.

Since the largest laxity in elbow specimens following ligament dissection was observed in elbow mid-flexion, this might be the best position for testing ligament integrity clinically.

Because of biomechanical disadvantages the load on the elbow joint can be heavy during flexion and extension, where the forces induced by the muscles are much higher than the external load applied to the hand. The contribution from the individual muscles to the induced force is influenced by the position of the elbow.

Q&A

1. What is the carrying angle?—It is defined as the angle between the long axis of the forearm relative to the long axis of the upper arm seen in full extension and disappeared in full flexion. This phenomenon is caused by the abducted hinge axis.
2. What is the primary elbow constraint of the MCL?—The MCL gives elbow constraint to forced valgus and internal rotation.
3. What is the primary constraint to posterolateral elbow joint instability?—The LCL that gives elbow constraint to forced varus and forced external rotation.
4. Why is the Terrible Triad of the elbow a potential clinical disaster?—The terrible triad is defined as concomitant elbow joint dislocation, with well documented bilateral ligament injury, and combined radial head and coronoid process fracture. This situation is a combination of total injury of the stabilizing ligaments and the axial stabilizers. Treatment requires a minimum of reconstruction of one of the axial stabilizers, preferentially the radial head and either LCL reconstruction or MCL and LCL reconstruction if the cornoid process and not the radial head is reconstructed.
5. Why is the elbow a load bearing joint?—Because of biomechanical disadvantages including the large distance from the axis of rotation to the insertion of the tendons of the major elbow muscles.

References

1. Jawa A, Jupiter JB, Ring D. Pathogenesis and classification of elbow stiffness. In: Stanley D, Trail I, editors. Operative elbow surgery. Edinburgh: Churchill Livingstone, Elsevier; 2012. p. 409–16.
2. Kapandji IA. The physiology of the joints. 5th ed. Edinburgh: Churchill Livingstone; 1982.
3. Zuckerman JD, Matsen FA. Biomechanics of the elbow. In: Nordin M, Frankel VH, editors. Basic biomechanics of the musculoskeletal system. 2nd ed. Philadelphia: Lea & Febiger; 1989. p. 249–61.
4. American Academy of Orthopaedic Surgeons. Joint and recording. Edinburgh: Churchill Livingstone; 1966.
5. Amis AA. Biomechanics of the elbow, Chap. 3. In: Stanley D, Trail I, editors. Operative elbow surgery. Edinburgh: Churchill Livingstone, Elsevier; 2012. p. 29–44.
6. Morrey BF, Askew LJ, Chao EY. A biomechanical study of normal functional elbow motion. JBJS (Am). 1981;63:872–7.
7. Amis AA, Dowson D, Wright V, et al. An examination of the elbow articulation with particular reference to the variation in the carrying angle. Eng Med. 1977;6:76–80.
8. Leonello DT, Galley IJ, Bain GI, et al. Brachialis muscle anatomy. A study in cadavers. J Bone Joint Surg Am. 2007;89:1293–7.
9. Stroyan M, Wilk KE. The functional anatomy of the elbow complex. J Orthop Sports Phys Ther. 1993;17:279–88.
10. Basmajian JV, Latif A. Integrated actions and functions of the chief flexors of the elbow. J Bone Joint Surg. 1957;39A:1106–18.
11. Madsen M, Marx RG, Millett PJ, et al. Surgical anatomy of the tricpes brachii tendon. Am J Sports Med. 2006;34:1839–43.
12. Thomas SJ, Yakin DE, Parry BR, et al. The anatomical relationship between the posterior interossseous nerve and the supinator muscle. J Hand Surg Am. 2000;25:936–41.
13. An KN, Hui FC, Morrey BF, et al. Muscles across the elbow joint. A biomechanical analysis. J Biomechan. 1981;14:659–69.
14. Basmajian JV, Travill A. Electromyography of the pronator muscles in the forearm. Anat Rec. 1961;139:45–9.
15. Olsen BS. Pathogenesis of chronic elbow instability, Chap. 25. In: Stanley D, Trail I, editors. Operative elbow surgery. Edinburgh: Churchill Livingstone, Elsevier; 2012. p. 369–83.
16. Morrey BF, Tanaka S, An KN. Valgus stability of the elbow: a definition of primary and secondary constraints. Clin Orthop Relat Res. 1991;265:187–95.
17. Jensen SL, Olsen BS, Søjbjerg JO. Elbow joint kinematics after excision of the radial head. J Shoulder Elbow Surg. 1999;8:238–41.

18. Jensen SL, Deutch SR, Olsen BS, Søjbjerg JO, Sneppen O. Laxity of the elbow after experimental excision of the radial head and division of the medial collateral ligament. J Bone Joint Surg Br. 2003;85B:1006–10.

19. Jensen SL, Olsen BS, Tyrdal S, Søjbjerg JO, Sneppen O. Elbow joint laxity after experimental radial head excision and lateral collateral ligament rupture. J Shoulder Elbow Surg. 2005;14:78–84.

20. Beingessner DM, Dunning CE, Gordon KD, Johnson JA, King GJ. The effect of radial head fracture size on elbow kinematics and stability. J Orthop Res. 2005;23:210–7.

21. Jensen SL, Olsen BS, Seki A, Søjbjerg JO, Sneppen O. Radiohumeral stability to forced translation. An experimental analysis of the bony constraint. J Shoulder Elbow Surg. 2002;11:158–65.

22. Deutch SR, Jensen SL, Tyrdal S, Olsen BS, Sneppen O. Elbow joint stability following experimental osteo-ligamentous injury and reconstruction. J Shoulder Elbow Surg. 2003;12:466–71.

23. Morrey BF, O'Driscoll SW. Elbow dislocation and complex instability of the elbow. In: Morrey BF, Sanchez-Sotello J, editors. The elbow and its disorders. 4th ed. Philadelphia: Saunders, Elsevier; 2008. p. 436–62.

24. Hotchkiss RN. Fractures and dislocations of the elbow. In: Rockwood CA, Green DP, editors. Rockwood and Green's fractures in adults. Philadelphia: Lippincott-Raven; 1996. p. 929–1024.

25. Beigenessner DM, Dunning CE, Stacpoole RA, Johnson JA, King GJ. The effect of coronoid fractures on elbow kinematics and stability. Clin Biomechanic. 2007;22:183–90.

26. Morrey BF, An KN. Stability of the elbow: osseous constraints. J Shoulder Elbow Surg. 2005;14-S:174S–8S.

27. Pollock JW, Brownhill J, Ferreira L, McDonald CP, Johnson J, King G. The effect of anteromedial facet fractures of the coronoid and lateral collateral ligament injury on elbow stability and kinematics. J Bone Joint Surg Am. 2009:1448–58.

28. O'Driscoll SW, Jupiter JB, Cohen MS, Ring D, McKee MD. Difficult elbow fractures: pearls and pitfalls. Instr Course Lect. 2003:113–34.

29. Regan W, Morrey B. Fractures of the coronoid process of the ulna. J Bone Joint Surg Am. 1989:1348–54.

30. Sanchez-Sotelo J, O'Driscoll SW, Morrey BF. Medial oblique compression fracture of the coronoid process of the ulna. J Shoulder Elbow Surg. 2005:60–4.

31. An KN, Morrey BF, Chao EY. The effects of partial removal of proximal ulna on elbow constraint. Clin Orthop Relat Res. 1986;209:270–9.

32. Kamineni S, Hirahara H, Pomianovski S, Neal PG, O'Driscoll SW, ElAttrache N, An KN, Morrey BF. Partial posteromedial olecranon resection: a kinematic study. J Bone Joint Surg Am. 2003;85-A:1005–11.

33. Dunning CE, Zarzour ZD, Patterson SD, Johnson JA, King GJ. Muscle forces and pronation stabilize the lateral ligament deficient elbow. Clin Orthop Relat Res. 2001;388:118–24.

34. Seiber K, Gupta R, McGarry MH, Safran MR, Lee TQ. The role of the elbow musculature, forearm rotation and elbow flexion in elbow stability: an in vitro study. J Shoulder Elbow Surg. 2009;18:260–8.

35. Josefsson PO, Johnell O, Wendeberg B. Ligamentous injuries in dislocations of the elbow joint. Clin Orthop Relat Res. 1987;221:221–5.

36. Morrey BF, An KN. Articular and ligamentous contributions to the stability of the elbow joint. Am J Sports Med. 1983;11:315–9.

37. Nielsen KK, Olsen BS. No stabilizing effect of the elbow joint capsule. A kinematic study. Acta orthop Scand. 1999;70:6–8.

38. Deutch SR, Olsen BS, Jensen SL, Tyrdal S, Sneppen O. Ligamentous and capsular restraints to experimental posterior elbow joint dislocation. Scand J Med Sci Sports. 2003;13:311–6.

39. O'Driscoll SW, Morrey BF, Korinek S, An KN. Elbow subluxation and dislocation: a spectrum of instability. Clin Orthop Relat Res. 1992;280:186–97.

40. Regan WD, Korinek SL, Morrey BF, An KN. Biomechanical study of ligaments around the elbow joint. Clin Orthop Relat Res. 1991;271:170–9.

41. Floris S, Olsen BS, Dalstra M, Søjbjerg JO, Sneppen O. The medial collateral ligament of the elbow joint. Anatomy and kinematics. J Shoulder Elbow Surg. 1998;7:345–51.

42. Callaway GH, Field LD, Deng XH, Torzilli PA, O'Brien SJ, Altchek DW, Warren RF. Biomechanical evaluation of the medial collateral ligament of the elbow. J Bone Join Surg Am. 1997;79A:1223–31.

43. Safran MR, Baillargeon D. Soft-tissue stabilizers of the elbow. J Shoulder Elbow Surg. 2005;14-S:179S–85S.

44. Armstrong AD, Dunning CE, Faber KJ, Duck TR, Johnson JA, King GJ. Rehabilitation of medial collateral ligament deficient elbow: an in vitro biomechanical study. J Hand Surg. 2000;25:1051–7.

45. O'Driscoll SW, Horii E, Morrey BF, Carmichael SW. Anatomy of the ulnar part of the lateral collateral ligament of the elbow. Clin Anat. 1992;5:296–303.

46. Olsen BS, Vaesel MT, Søjbjerg JO, Helmig P, Sneppen O. Lateral collateral ligament of the elbow joint. Anatomy and kinematics. J Shoulder Elbow Surg. 1996;5:103–12.

47. Olsen BS, Søjbjerg JO, Dalstra M, Sneppen O. Kinematics of the lateral ligamentous constraints of the elbow joint. J Shoulder Elbow Surg. 1996;5:333–41.

48. Olsen BS, Søjbjerg JO, Nielsen KK, Vaesel MT, Dalstra M, Sneppen O. Posterolateral elbow joint instability. The basic kinematics. J Shoulder Elbow Surg. 1998;7:19–29.

49. Cohen MS, Hasting H. Rotatory instability of the elbow. The anatomy and role of the lateral stabilizers. J Bone Joint Surg Am. 1997;79A:225–33.

50. Dunning CE, Zarzour ZD, Patterson SD, Johnson JA, King GJ. Ligamentous stabilizers against

posterolateral rotatory instability of the elbow. J Bone
Joint Surg Am. 2001;83-A:1823–8.

51. O'Driscoll SW, Bell DF, Morrey BF. Posterolateral
rotatory instability of the elbow. J Bone Joint Surg
Am. 1991;73-A:440–6.

52. Messier RH, Duffy J, Litchman HM, et al. The electromyogram as a measure of tension in the human biceps
and trceps muscles. Int J Mech Sci. 1971;13:585–98.

53. Amis AA, Dawson D, Wright V. Elbow joint force
predictions for some strenuous isometric actions. J
Biomech. 1980;13:765–75.

54. Funk DA, An KN, Morrey BF, et al. Electromyographic
analysis of muscles across the elbow joint. J Orthop
Res. 1987;5:529–38.

55. Stevens A, Stijns H, Reybrouck T, et al. A polyelec-
tromyographical study of the arm muscles at gradual
isometric loading. Electromyogr Clin Neurophysiol.
1973;13:465–76.

56. Basmajian JV. Recent advances in the functional anatomy of the upper limb. Am J Phys Med. 1969;48:165.

57. Travell AA. Electromyographic study of the extensor
apparatus of the forearm. Anat Rec. 1962;144:373–6.

58. Haugstvedt JR, Berger RA, Bjerglund LJ. A mechanical study of the moment-forces of the supinators
and pronators of the forearm. Acta Orthop Scand.
2001;72:629–34.

Elbow Injuries in the Throwing Athlete

4

Ann-Maria Byrne and Roger van Riet

Contents

Key Learning Points

1. Medial elbow pain in the throwing athlete can arise from multiple pathologies
2. Overuse injuries arise from recurrent valgus loading of the medial elbow
3. Acute injuries can result in MCL avulsion from the humeral or ulnar insertions
4. MCL insufficiency can be a career-changing injury in elite throwing athletes
5. MCL reconstructive surgery is reserved for throwing athletes with a complete MCL tear or those with partial tears that have failed rehabilitation
6. Non-throwing athletes who continue to be symptomatic after rehabilitation may benefit from MCL reconstruction.

A.-M. Byrne
Sport Surgery Clinic, Dublin, Ireland
e-mail: ambyrneadmin@sportssurgeryclinic.com

R. van Riet (✉)
AZ Monica, Antwerp, Belgium

University Hospital Antwerp, Antwerp, Belgium
e-mail: drrogervanriet@azmonica.be

4.1 Introduction

In recent years, there has been a considerable rise in the number of athletes participating in overhead throwing sports. This rise has brought a concurrent increase in the incidence of elbow injuries, resulting in distinctive injury patterns specific to the throwing athlete. Waris first described a throwing injury to the ulnar collateral ligament in javelin throwers in 1946 [1]. Since then, research on elbow injuries in the throwing athlete has been focused on baseball pitchers, where the elbow is subjected to significant valgus stresses during throwing actions, and the forces generated are concentrated mainly at the medial structures of the elbow. Power grip in racquet sports, weight bearing in gymnastics and weight-lifting, have also been implicated in medial elbow symptoms [2]. Medial elbow symptoms represent 97% of all elbow problems in baseball players [3], however, similar elbow complaints arise in athletes participating in javelin, tennis, handball, volleyball and water polo.

Medial elbow problems in the throwing athlete can encompass a broad spectrum of pathology due to the tensile forces applied to the medial stabilising structures, combined with lateral compartment compression and posterior shear forces [4]. Repetitive valgus stresses may lead to a selection of chronic overuse problems, but athletes can also present with acute and acute-on-chronic injuries. Just some of the injuries encountered in the throwing elbow include ulnar collateral ligament tears, ulnar neuritis, flexor-pronator tendinopathy/tears, medial epicondyle apophysitis/avulsion, and valgus extension overload syndrome [5–8]. In treating athletes who participate in overhead throwing sports, an understanding of functional elbow anatomy and the biomechanics of throwing are essential in the diagnosis and management of these unique elbow injuries.

4.2 Anatomy

The elbow joint is a modified hinge and the bony anatomy of the ulnohumeral articulation provides primary static stability at the extremes of motion, at less than 20° and beyond 120° of flexion [4, 7]. Both static and dynamic stability are required in the intervening 100°, which is the primary arc of motion used during overhead throwing activities [4, 9]. The bony configuration of the elbow provides approximately 50% of overall stability, mainly against varus stress in the extended elbow. Dynamic stability is provided by the anterior capsule of the elbow joint and the medial and lateral collateral ligament complexes [3]. In full extension, valgus stability is provided by osseous constraints, the medial collateral ligament (MCL) complex, and the anterior capsule. At 90° of flexion, the anterior capsule becomes lax and the MCL assumes a greater role, providing 54% of the stabilising force against valgus stresses [9, 10].

The MCL complex is comprised of three bundles, the anterior and posterior bundles and a variable oblique transverse bundle (Fig. 4.1) [4].

The anterior bundle consists of parallel fibres arising from the undersurface of the medial epicondyle, inserting onto the sublime tubercle of the ulna. It acts as the primary restraint to valgus stress to the elbow from 30° to 120° of flexion [11]. Sequential tightening occurs within the anterior bundle fibres, moving from anterior to posterior with elbow flexion [3]. Callaway et al. [12] characterised the bundle fibres as acting in a reciprocal manner by stabilising the elbow

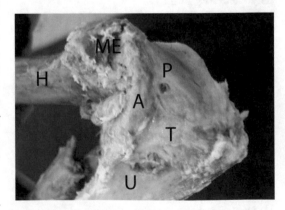

Fig. 4.1 Cadaveric dissection of the medial side of the elbow. Three parts of the Medial Collateral Ligament complex can be distinguished. *H* humerus, *U* ulna, *ME* medial epicondyle, *A* anterior band of the MCL, *P* posterior band, *T* transverse band (Copyright of MoRe Foundation)

throughout the flexion-extension arc. They found the anterior bundle to act as the primary stabiliser from 30° to 90°, while both bands acted together to stabilise the elbow at 120° of flexion. As a thickening of the joint capsule, the posterior bundle alone adds little to withstand valgus stresses, however, at 30° of flexion it acts as a secondary stabiliser, and becomes functionally more important between 60° and full flexion [3, 12].

4.3 Biomechanics of MCL Injury During Throwing

Different sporting activities require an assortment of throwing techniques, however, the overall basic throwing action is similar. The throwing motion generates significant valgus and extension stress to the elbow. Much of the published research in this area has been focused on throwing injuries in baseball pitchers, and their overhead throwing motion has been divided into six stages: (1) windup, (2) early cocking, (3) late cocking, (4) acceleration, (5) deceleration, and (6) follow through [13, 14]. During the late cocking and acceleration phases, the MCL complex of the elbow experiences tremendous valgus stresses. Tensile forces approaching the point of failure of the anterior bundle have been reported during the acceleration phase of high velocity throwing [11, 13]. The anterior bundle is more susceptible to injury by valgus stress to the extended elbow, while the posterior bundle is more vulnerable with elbow flexion [3, 11, 12, 14]. Biomechanical studies have demonstrated the ultimate load to failure of the native anterior bundle in resisting valgus torque to be 34 Nm [15], while the potential valgus stresses on the MCL during overhead throwing have been found to approach 35 Nm [13]. Fleisig et al. [13] also demonstrated valgus forces as high as 64 Nm to the elbow itself during late cocking and early acceleration, with lateral radiocapitellar compressive forces of 500 N as the elbow moves from 110° to 20° of flexion with velocities as high as 3000° per second.

The anterior bundle of the MCL complex bears the majority of these valgus forces. Repetitive valgus tensile loads associated with poor throw-

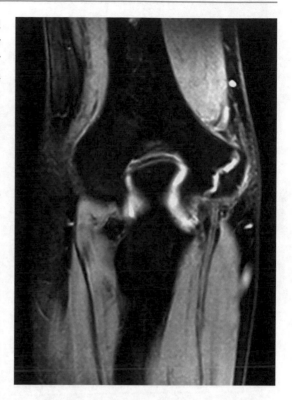

Fig. 4.2 Magnetic Resonance Image of a medial epicondyle apophysitis in a skeletally immature athlete (Copyright of MoRe Foundation)

ing technique, may lead to anterior bundle attenuation and eventually even rupture [4, 16]. Simultaneous elbow extension during the throwing motion can also cause the MCL to undergo significant bending stresses that generate destructive internal shearing stresses between the fibres of the ligament itself [17]. Secondary supporting structures on the medial side of the elbow may be stretched due to valgus laxity, resulting in flexor-pronator mass tendonopathy, ulnar neuritis, or medial epicondyle apophysitis in the skeletally immature patient [4, 9] (Fig. 4.2).

During extension in the follow-through phase of throwing, shear forces on the posterior compartment may produce posteriomedial olecranon osteophytes, with a corresponding olecranon fossa "kissing lesion" (Fig. 4.3). Subsequent overload in the lateral compartment of the elbow leads to abnormal compressive forces across the radiocapitellar articulation, resulting in chondromalacia, osteophyte and loose body formation.

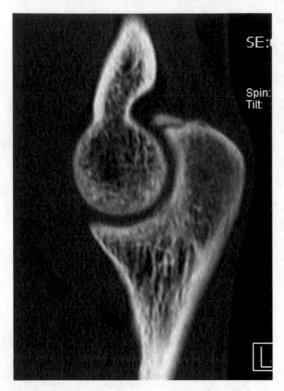

Fig. 4.3 CT scan of the elbow showing a fractured osteophyte at the tip of the olecranon (Copyright of MoRe Foundation)

This constellation of findings has been termed the "valgus extension overload syndrome' (VEOS) and is the basic model behind most common elbow injuries in the throwing athlete [4, 8, 18].

4.4 History and Examination

In the assessment of elbow problems in athletes, valuable information will be obtained with a thorough history and physical examination. Details on the events preceding the injury should be recorded, including previous injuries, prodromal symptoms, and changes in training regimens. The athlete may report an acute episode of medial elbow pain, with or without a "popping' sensation, during a throwing motion, and may be unable to continue throwing [3]. However, the more common history encountered is of an insidious onset of pain with gradual loss of ball control and reduction of peak velocities, throwing dis-

tance and endurance [17, 19, 20]. The exact site of pain, with the phase of throwing during which pain is experienced, should be noted. Pain usually reaches maximal intensity during the late cocking and early acceleration phases, but with VEOS, athletes may report posteromedial pain during deceleration due to osteophyte impingement [20]. Medial joint opening or instability symptoms may also be a feature [21], and ulnar nerve symptoms at rest or during throwing should be recorded.

Physical examination of the elbow begins systematically with inspection of the joint in its resting position. Ecchymosis may be seen with fractures, tendon or acute ligament ruptures or elbow dislocations (Fig. 4.4).

Fullness in the soft spot, the area triangulated by the lateral epicondyle, the tip of the olecranon and the radial head, may indicate the presence of synovitis or a joint effusion. With an acute elbow joint effusion, the athlete may hold the elbow flexed to 70°, the position of comfort, to accommodate increased capsular distention. The carrying angle is the angle formed by a line drawn along the humeral axis and a second line along the forearm axis: the normal valgus carrying angle in men and women is 11° and 13°, respectively. It is not unusual to see an increased valgus carrying angle in the throwing elbow as a result of adaptation to repetitive stress, and valgus angles of more than 15° have been reported in professional throwers [4, 22].

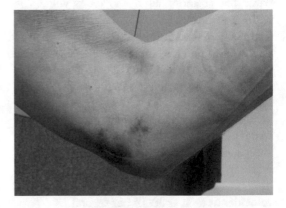

Fig. 4.4 Clinical photograph of the medial side of the elbow following an elbow dislocation. Echymosis is indicative of a medial collateral ligament injury (Copyright of MoRe Foundation)

Palpation of the bony landmarks should be performed, paying particular attention to the medial side of the elbow and the posteromedial olecranon. Athletes with MCL injuries commonly complain of pain over the ulnar insertion onto the sublime tubercle. In the skeletally immature athlete, medial epicondylar pain may be due to a growth plate injury or avulsion fracture. Active and passive range of motion should then be assessed, and any pain, crepitus, locking or loss of motion should be documented. The end-point in extension is important to note in the throwing elbow [4]. Up to 50% of professional throwers demonstrate elbow flexion contractures that may not be indicative of pathology. However, an osseus block to terminal extension may be due to osteophyte or loose body formation [8, 22].

The ulnar nerve can be traumatised by relatively small degrees of valgus instability, and is vulnerable in its position in the cubital tunnel along the posterior aspect of the medial epicondyle [7]. The nerve should be checked for subluxation out of the cubital tunnel. Usually the unstable ulnar nerve dislocates anterior to the medial epicondyle when the elbow is moved from extension to flexion [23]. The ulnar nerve is examined for instability during eccentric loading of the triceps. A distal muscle belly can actively force the ulnar nerve out of its groove, causing a subluxation or a painful snap (Fig. 4.5). Tinel's sign is elicited with percussion along the nerve, causing paraesthesia of the ring and small fin-

gers. The distal medial aspect of the triceps tendon should also be palpated; as anomalous bands of the distal triceps insertion have been described as a cause of ulnar nerve impingement. This can also produce a snapping sensation as they move across the medial epicondyle [24].

4.4.1 Special Tests

Valgus stress testing is performed to evaluate the integrity of the anterior bundle of the MCL. To unlock the ulnohumeral articulation, testing is performed at 20°–30° elbow flexion with the forearm pronated [25]. O'Driscoll et al. [26] advised that forearm pronation prevents subtle posterolateral instability from mimicking medial laxity. In the supine position, the examiner stabilises the right humerus with the left hand just above the humeral condyles and applies a valgus moment with the right hand while holding the patient's pronated forearm. The ilpsilateral elbow is also tested for pain and medial opening. In the throwing elbow, medial instability may be very subtle even with a significant MCL injury, and it has been shown that complete sectioning of the anterior bundle of the MCL only increases medial opening by 1–2 mm [7, 27].

The "milking maneuver" described by Veltri et al. [28], is a provocative test that applies a valgus stress preferentially to the anterior bundle of the MCL. The examiner grasps the thumb on the affected side, with the arm in 90° of shoulder abduction and 90° elbow flexion, representing the cocked phase of throwing. A valgus stress is then applied by pulling down on the thumb, in a similar manner to pulling down on the teats when milking a cow, from which the test derives its name. Reproduction of pain indicates a positive test.

The "moving valgus stress" test was described by O'Driscoll et al. [17]. The patient is positioned upright with the shoulder abducted to 90°. A valgus stress is applied to the forearm until the shoulder reaches maximum external rotation. At maximal elbow flexion, the elbow is rapidly extended to 30°, while maintaining a constant

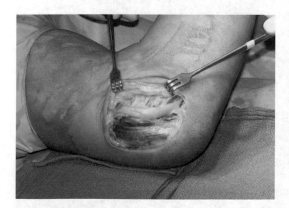

Fig. 4.5 A distal triceps muscle belly causing a symptomatic dislocation of the ulnar nerve, can be seen in this patient (Copyright of MoRe Foundation)

valgus force. A positive result requires two conditions to be satisfied: firstly, pain elicited must be similar to that during the act of throwing; and secondly, maximal pain must occur during the position of late cocking (120° elbow flexion) and early acceleration (30° elbow flexion). The specific angle of maximum pain is referred to as the shear angle, whereas the total arc of motion that is painful is referred to as the shear range. The investigators have reported a positive test to have 100% sensitivity and 75% specificity for MCL tears.

With the valgus extension overload test, the examiner forces the flexed elbow into full extension while applying a valgus stress [8]. This manoeuvre attempts to reproduce the posteromedial pain of impingement as the olecranon tip engages against the medial wall of the olecranon fossa. A positive test indicates the presence of a posteromedial olecranon osteophyte or overgrowth of the olecranon fossa.

4.5   Imaging Studies

There has been significant debate regarding the diagnostic accuracy of imaging studies regarding MCL pathology, and all imaging must be correlated with history and clinical examination. Plain radiographs may demonstrate changes consistent with chronic instability, such as calcification or ossification of the MCL (Fig. 4.6). Loose bodies, osteophytes and radiocapitellar pathology may also be seen.

Valgus stress radiographs can be used to confirm instability, particularly in patients with equivocal clinical findings. Stress radiography of the dominant elbow in baseball players with MCL injuries showed it to have 0.4 mm greater opening compared with the 'non-throwing' arm, and openings of 0.6 mm greater were found with full-thickness MCL tears [29]. Interestingly, baseball players with a partial MCL tear had decreased laxity on valgus stress (0.1 mm) [29]. Dynamic

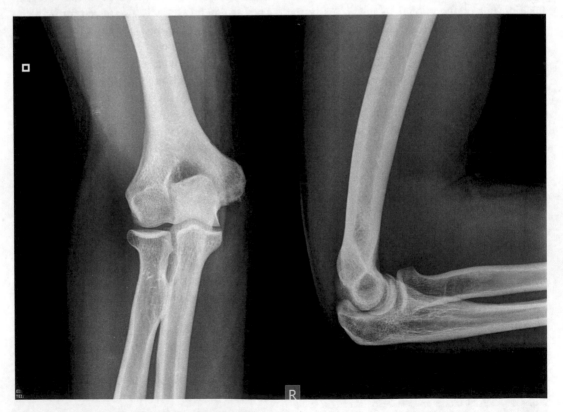

Fig. 4.6 Plain radiographic anteroposterior and lateral views of the elbow, showing calcification of the medial epicondyle as an indirect sign of chronic instability (Copyright of MoRe Foundation)

ultrasonography and fluoroscopic valgus test under anaesthesia have also been described as assisting in the diagnosis of instability and MCL insufficiency [30–32]. Traditionally, medial joint opening greater than 3 mm is consistent with instability [14, 33].

Magnetic resonance imaging (MRI) can be a valuable tool in the assessment of MCL tears, osteochondral injuries, olecranon osteophytes, loose bodies and sites of neurologic compression (Fig. 4.7).

One series reported MRI without arthrography to have 57% sensitivity and 100% specificity in detecting full thickness MCL tears, however, only detected partial tears in 14% of patients [34]. The addition of contrast gives improved visualisation of the undersurface of the MCL for diagnosis of partial tears [35, 36]. Saline-enhanced MR Arthrograms of the elbow were performed by Schwartz et al. [37] by injecting into the joint through the lateral soft spot. They found saline extravasation through the MCL to be diagnostic of full-thickness injury, and reported 92% sensitivity and 100% specificity in the diagnosis of ulnar collateral ligament tears. Sensitivity was higher for complete tears (95%) than for partial tears (86%).

Computed tomography (CT) scans are very helpful in patients where associated bony lesions

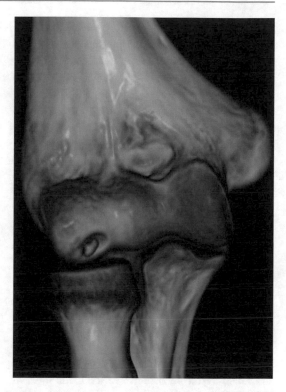

Fig. 4.8 3D CT scan showing sequelae of osteochondritis dissecans caused by valgus extension overload syndrome prevalent in throwing athletes (Copyright of MoRe Foundation)

such as osteochondirits dissecans (Fig. 4.8), loose bodies or osteophyte formation are suspected (Fig. 4.3). CT arthrography has been shown by Timmerman et al. [34] to demonstrate a 'T-sign' that represents an undersurface tear of the MCL. This undersurface tear allows dye to leak around the detached distal insertion but remains ultimately contained within the superficial layer of the ligament and capsule. They reported sensitivity of 86% and specificity of 91% for undersurface MCL tears in a population of baseball players. We prefer to use MRI to evaluate the soft tissue in these patients and reserve CT scanning for bony abnormalities.

4.6 Treatment Options

Once a diagnosis is confirmed, treatment should be customised to the athlete's functional demands and level of impairment. Informed discussion

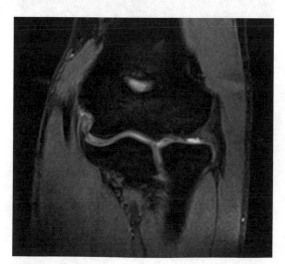

Fig. 4.7 MRI scan of the elbow, showing a full thickness tear of the medial collateral ligament (Copyright of MoRe Foundation)

between the athlete and treating physician or surgeon will assess the appropriate care pathway, whether that is conservative management, or surgery followed by rehabilitation. It is important to include trainers, coaches and potentially other supporting staff in the discussion to optimise a multidisciplinary approach. Non-operative treatment begins with a period of rest from throwing [38, 39]. Patients progress through a programme promoting elbow range of motion, flexor-pronator strengthening, leading to retraining in throwing mechanics at approximately 3 months [21, 40]. Following this period of rest and physiotherapy, if the athlete is asymptomatic and has a normal exam, then return to throwing with optimising throwing mechanics, is acceptable [38]. Jobe (unpublished data, 1992) described a protocol of two cycles of 3 months' rest from throwing and treatment with rehabilitation exercises [41]. No rates of return to play after this nonoperative treatment were reported. Rettig et al. [41] demonstrated a 42% return to the same level of play with an average return at 24.5 weeks with non-operative management in baseball pitchers with MCL injuries. They found no difference in prognosis between athletes with acute or insidious onset of symptoms, nor did they find a relationship between the age of the athlete at the time of onset of symptoms and the outcome of non-operative treatment. Adjuvant treatments used have included phonophoresis, iontophoresis, and electrical stimulation [21].

Optimising technique is even more important in patients with a valgus overload syndrome, without an MCL tear. Without this, the risk of recurrent symptoms is extremely high, even if conservative treatment is successful initially.

Elbow arthroscopy can play a role in diagnosing MCL insufficiency with the elbow arthroscopic valgus instability test, described by Field and Altchek [27]. When viewed from the anterolateral portal, a valgus stress is applied to the elbow, which is flexed between 60° and 75° with the forearm in pronation. A positive result will demonstrate opening of the ulnohumeral articulation of greater than 1 mm (Fig. 4.9).

Arthroscopy may also have a role in treating synchronous intra-articular pathology as seen in

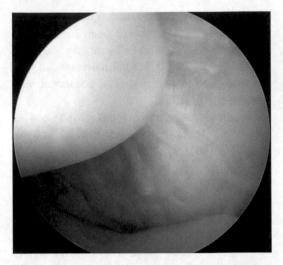

Fig. 4.9 Arthroscopic valgus stress view of the ulnar gutter and medial ulnohumeral joint space in a patient with a complete insufficiency of the medial collateral ligament complex (Copyright of MoRe Foundation)

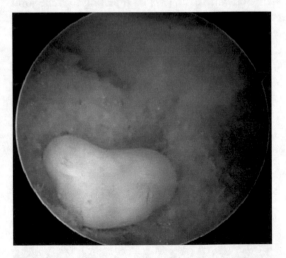

Fig. 4.10 Arthroscopic removal of a loose body (Copyright of MoRe Foundation)

the valgus extension overload syndrome [8, 9]. Success in the arthroscopic management of many pathologies of the thrower's elbow have been reported, including osteophyte debridement for posteromedial impingement, loose body removal (Fig. 4.10), capsular release, treatment of osteochondritis dissecans (Fig. 4.8), and debridement for lateral epicondylitis [9].

Dodson et al. [19] performed routine arthroscopy in patients prior to reconstruction of the

MCL. They removed osteophytes from either the posteromedial olecranon or the coronoid process in 29% of cases, performed microfracture on cartilaginous defects in 9%, and removed loose bodies in 7%. A concern has arisen where excessive olecranon resection may lead to a loss of ulnohumeral constraint and thus increasing stresses on the MCL [5, 20, 42]. One study demonstrated that 25% of professional athletes who underwent debridement of posteromedial olecranon osteophytes developed iatrogenic valgus instability possibly contributing to MCL insufficiency. Kamineni et al. [42] reported on the amount of olecranon that can be safely resected, ranging from 3 to 8 mm. Failure to diagnose and treat osseous lesions in athletes with VEOS, will result in continued posteromedial pain from impingement of these osteophytes against the wall of the olecranon fossa and potential need for reoperation, even after a successful MCL reconstruction [8, 9, 19].

Indications for surgical MCL reconstruction require an accurate diagnosis with confirmatory history, physical exam, and imaging studies. Athletes with a diagnosis of MCL insufficiency who fail non-operative treatment, and those who wish to return to throwing, are candidates for surgical reconstruction. In an athlete with a history of acute onset of pain and confirmation of a complete tear on imaging studies, many surgeons would offer surgery within 2 weeks of injury [20]. Some athletes may be able to modify their sporting activities to reduce valgus loading of the elbow, making surgery unnecessary. The decision to suggest a surgical reconstruction is very difficult in high level athletes with a partial MCL tear and symptomatic VEOS, without bony abnormalities. Conservative treatment, including flexor-pronator group strengthening and a thorough analysis and adaptation of their technique are certainly the first choice. However, it is unknown how long conservative measures should be maintained before surgery would be indicated. A prolonged period of inactivity from their sport with an uncertain outcome of conservative treatment is problematic for these athletes and there is a lot of pressure on the athlete and the surgeon to perform a procedure that may ulti-

mately not be in the best interest of this particular patient. Contraindications to surgical management include patients with asymptomatic tears of the MCL [43]. Concomitant ulnohumeral or radiocapitellar arthritis is only a relative contraindication to surgical reconstruction, as this may decrease the chance of a successful outcome [41]. With ligament reconstruction, such patients may experience an exacerbation of joint pain [20].

Direct repair of the MCL is only indicated in cases of acute avulsion from the humeral origin or the coronoid insertion [3, 16, 43] (Fig. 4.11).

The direct repair may be reinforced with a tendon graft, creating a hybrid technique (Fig. 4.12). Most MCL reconstruction techniques involve a free tendon graft, usually placed in bone tunnels

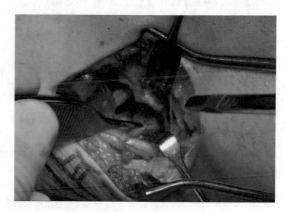

Fig. 4.11 Intra-operative view of the elbow showing a complete avulsion of the MCL (Copyright of MoRe Foundation)

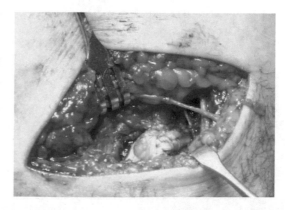

Fig. 4.12 Medial collateral reconstruction using a hybrid technique of repair and a tendon graft (Copyright of MoRe Foundation)

in the humerus and ulna. Graft options previously described include autologous and allograft palmaris longus tendon, plantaris tendon, hamstring tendons, and strips of Achilles or triceps tendon [3, 16, 43–45].

Jobe et al. [16] developed the original MCL reconstruction technique, which consisted of tendinous transection and reflection of the flexor-pronator mass, submuscular transposition of the ulnar nerve, and creation of humeral tunnels that penetrate the posterior humeral cortex. While this technique was successful in returning throwing athletes back to their pre-injury level, it was technically demanding and there was a high complication rate of up to 21%, most often with ulnar nerve problems [16, 39]. Since then, his technique has been modified to reduce the technical demands and reduce soft-tissue morbidity [40]. A muscle-splitting approach (Fig. 4.13) has been developed to avoid detachment of the flexor-pronator mass, with or without anterior subcutaneous transposition of the ulnar nerve [46].

To avoid subsequent ulnar nerve symptoms and the need for transposition, Hotchkiss [47] described his "over-the-top" approach, leaving the ulnar nerve in situ. Modifications of the original Jobe technique recommend that bone tunnels are directed anteriorly on the humeral epicondyle to avoid the risk of ulnar nerve injury, while the graft is passed in a figure-of-eight fashion. Other changes in bone tunnel configuration have been developed, the number of bone tunnels have been

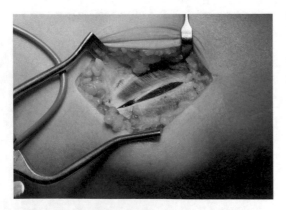

Fig. 4.13 Muscle splitting approach decreases soft-tissue dissection and co-morbidity involved with other approaches (Copyright of MoRe Foundation)

reduced to facilitate better graft tensioning and to avoid the risk of iatrogenic fracture [40, 48, 49]. Several methods of graft fixation have been described, including transosseus figure-of-eight reconstruction, docking technique, docking technique employing additional strands, hybrid interference screw fixation, and EndoButton fixation [16, 42, 44, 48, 49].

Following surgical reconstruction, the elbow is immobilised in a splint for 24 hours. We then protect the reconstruction using a dynamic elbow brace. Rehabilitation commences immediately with active wrist, elbow, and shoulder range-of-motion exercises. The brace allows full flexion and extension is blocked to 60° for the first 2 weeks. This is increased to 30° at 2 weeks and full extension in the brace is allowed from weeks 4–6 postoperatively. Strengthening exercises also start 4–6 weeks postoperatively. Valgus stress should be avoided until 4 months postoperatively, at which time the patient may begin a supervised throwing programme consisting of gradually increasing ball toss distances for longer periods of time. At 6 months, the patient may throw lightly from the windup [40]. Throwing in competition is permitted at 1 year, if the shoulder, elbow, and forearm are pain free during throwing and if full strength and motion has returned [40].

Clinical outcomes for MCL reconstruction have been variable with 68–93% having good to excellent results [39]. Later studies have shown improvements on the original Jobe technique with better results, often attributed to reduced dissection of the flexor-pronator mass, and better handling of the ulnar nerve [40]. Thompson et al. [46] reported on 93% of patients undergoing MCL reconstruction with excellent results at 2-year follow-up. Azar et al. [44] reported on 78 throwing athletes who underwent MCL reconstruction with submuscular ulnar nerve transposition. Of the 59 patients available for follow-up at 12–72 months, 81% returned to the same or higher level of competition. Rohrbough et al. [49] reported on 36 patients where they utilised the docking technique. At average follow-up of 3.3 years, 92% returned to or improved their previous level of competition for at least 1 year. Jiang and Leland [50] recently reported on 41 major league baseball pitchers. Three players (7%) needed a revision and eight players did not return to the major league level (20%). Statistical performance measurements showed that the other players returned to their pre-injury level after 1-year post surgery. Even velocity of pitching returned to pre-injury level. Erickson et al. [51] analysed the statistical performance measurements of 179 major league baseball pitchers. They found a significant decrease in performance in the year before surgery, which improved significantly and predictably post-surgery. A total of 83% were able to return to play in the major league, with a later revision rate of 3.9%. [51]. Sparse literature is available on return to play following revision MCL reconstruction. Although approximately 75% are able to return to major league baseball, the pitch workload is clearly decreased with pitchers only reaching 35–50% of their pre-injury throwing activity [52].

4.7   Summary

The incidence of medial sided injuries from overhead sports has risen in recent years. Medial elbow symptoms in the throwing athlete can arise from multiple pathologies. There is a spectrum of injuries, from an acute strain or rupture of the MCL to chronic valgus overload syndrome, leading to arthritis and MCL insufficiency. The most common constellation of symptoms occurs with Valgus Extension Overload Syndrome. Associated MCL insufficiency is potentially a career-changing injury in overhead throwing athletes. The diagnosis is mainly clinical with several specific tests that can be used. Radiographic imaging, CT and MRI may be used to confirm the diagnosis, but are particularly helpful in diagnosing associated pathology such as cartilage lesions, osteophytes or loose bodies.

Treatment options depend on the sport, and the remaining ambition of the athlete. Management of medial elbow symptoms in the non-throwing athlete and low-demand patients may be treated non-operatively. Conservative treatment will initially include rest and anti-inflammatory measures, followed by strengthening exercises and progressive

loading of the elbow. A thorough analysis and improvement of technique, where possible, are imperative for conservative treatment to be successful. Results of conservative treatment may be disappointing in the face of degenerative changes in the elbow joint. If present, loose bodies or osteophytes should be removed in conjunction with conservative measures described. This can best be done arthroscopically. Elbow arthroscopy has the added benefit that the MCL can be evaluated directly. Medial opening of the joint space by more than 1 mm is indicative of an insufficiency of the MCL.

Direct repair of the acutely avulsed MCL may be indicated in select patients, but as the quality of the ligament is usually decreased from chronic overuse, this may not be strong enough and a reconstruction or hybrid technique is often indicated. Surgical reconstruction of the MCL is warranted for throwing athletes with complete MCL tears or those with partial tears that have failed rehabilitation, in addition to non-throwing athletes who are still symptomatic following rehabilitation or direct repair. Evolution of Jobe's original MCL reconstruction technique over the past 30 years has seen modifications such as the docking technique, interference screw fixation, and use of suture anchors. However, successful outcomes following MCL reconstruction hinge on decreased dissection of the flexor-pronator mass, decreased handling of the ulnar nerve, and recognition and treatment of associated medial and intra-articular elbow pathologies.

Q&A
1. How are MCL injuries best diagnosed

Clinical examination is the mainstay of diagnosing MCL injuries. Radiographs, CT or MRI will aid in the diagnosis but are mainly important in discovering associated pathology.

2. How are MCL injuries managed?

Sports technique (e.g. throwing, tennis serve) needs to be an integral part of conservative treatment, before, or rehabilitation, after, surgery.

Arthroscopy is a useful tool in the workup of the thrower's elbow and is imperative in the presence of loose bodies or osteophytes. If these measures do not provide relief then medial ligament reconstruction can be considered. The choice of graft and fixation of the graft can be left to the surgeon's preference as no significant clinical benefit has been shown in favour of one technique.

3. What are the risks in the management of MCL injuries?

Conservative treatment for an MCL tear is only successful in 42% of patients. A primary repair of an MCL tear may fail early in patients with pre-existing symptoms, due to decreased quality of the native ligament. Ulnar nerve symptoms are common preoperatively. Examine the ulnar nerve for compression or snapping as a release or transposition may be indicated. If MCL reconstruction is postponed too long, degenerative changes of the elbow will occur in many patients with chronic valgus laxity. This will negatively affect the result of treatment. Results of an MCL reconstruction are best in the absence of osteoarthritis.

References

1. Waris W. Elbow injuries of javelin-throwers. Acta Chir Scand. 1946;93:563.
2. Gregory B, Nyland J. Medial elbow injury in young throwing athletes. Musc Ligam Tendons J. 2013;3(2):91–100.
3. Chen FS, Rokito AS, Jobe FW. Medial elbow problems in the overhead-throwing athlete. JAAOS. 2001;9(2):99–113.
4. Cain EL, Dugas JR, Wolf RS, Andrews JR. Elbow injuries in throwing athletes: a current concepts review. Am J Sports Med. 2003;31(4):621–35.
5. Andrews JR, Timmerman LA. Outcome of elbow surgery in professional baseball players. Am J Sports Med. 1995;23:407–13.
6. Barnes DA, Tullos HS. An analysis of 100 symptomatic baseball players. Am J Sports Med. 1978;6:62–7.
7. Cain EL, Dugan JR. History and examination of the thrower's elbow. Clin Sports Med. 2004;23:553–66.
8. Wilson FD, Andrew JR, Blackburn TA, McCluskey G. Valgus extension overload in the pitching elbow. Am J Sports Med. 1983;11:83–8.
9. O'Holleran JD, Altchek DW. The Thrower's Elbow: arthroscopic treatment of valgus extension overload syndrome. HSSJ. 2006;2:83–93.
10. Morrey BF, An KN. Articular and ligamentous contributions to the stability of the elbow joint. Am J Sports Med. 1983;11:315–9.
11. Morrey BF, Tanaka S, An KN. Valgus stability of the elbow: a definition of primary and secondary constraints. Clin Orthop. 1991;265:187–95.
12. Callaway GH, Field LD, Deng XH, et al. Biomechanical evaluation of the Medial Collateral Ligament of the elbow. J Bone Joint Surg (Am). 1997;79:1223–31.
13. Fleisig GS, Andrews JR, Dillman CJ, et al. Kinetics of baseball pitching with implications about injury mechanisms. Am J Sports Med. 1995;23:233–9.
14. Jobe FW, Kvitne RS. Elbow instability in the athlete. Instr Course Lect. 1991;40:17–23.
15. Admad CS, Lee TQ, ElAttrache NS. Biomechanical evaluation of a new ulnar collateral ligament reconstruction technique with interference screw fixation. Am J Sports Med. 2003;31:332–7.
16. Jobe FW, Stark H, Lombardo SJ. Reconstruction of the ulnar collateral ligament in athletes. J Bone Joint Surg Am. 1986;68:1158–63.
17. O'Driscoll SW, Lawton RL, Smith AM. The moving valgus stress test for medial collateral ligament tears of the elbow. Am J Sports Med. 2005;33:231–9.
18. Miller CD, Savoie FH III. Valgus extension injuries of the elbow in the throwing athlete. J Am Acad Orthop Surg. 1994;2:261–9.
19. Dodson CC, Thomas A, Dines JS, et al. Medial ulnar collateral ligament reconstruction in throwing athletes. Am J Sports Med. 2006;34:1926–32.
20. Wong AS, Baratz ME. Sports injuries of the elbow. In: Stanley D, Trail IA, editors. Operative elbow surgery: Elsevier; 2012. p. 494–508.
21. Cicotti MG, Jobe FW. Medial collateral ligament instability and ulnar neuritis in the athlete's elbow. AAOS Instruct Course Lect. 1999;48:383–91.
22. King JW, Brelsford HJ, Tullos HS. Analysis of the pitching arm of the professional baseball pitcher. Clin Orthop. 1969;67:116–23.
23. Del Pizzo W, Jobe FW, Norwood L. Ulnar nerve entrapment syndrome in baseball players. Am J Sports Med. 1977;5:182–5.
24. Spinner RJ, Goldner RD. Snapping of the medal head of the triceps and recurrent dislocation of the ulnar nerve. J Bone joint Surg. 1998;80A:239–47.
25. Norwood LA, Shook JA, Andrews JR. Acute medial elbow ruptures. Am J Sports Med. 1981;9:16–9.
26. O'Driscoll SW, Bell DF, Morrey BF. Posterolateral rotatory instability of the elbow. J Bone Joint Surg. 1991;73A:440–6.
27. Field LD, Altchek DW. Evaluation of the arthroscopic valgus instability test of the elbow. Am J Sports Med. 1996;24:177–81.
28. Veltri DM, O'Brien SJ, Field LD, et al. The milking maneuver: a new test to evaluate the MCL of the elbow in the throwing athlete. In: Programs and abstracts of the 10th open meeting of the American Shoulder and Elbow Surgeons. Rosemont, IL: American Academy of Orthopaedic Surgeons; 1994.

29. Bruce JR, Hess R, Joyner P, Andrews JR. How much valgus instability can be expected with ulnar collateral ligament (UCL) injuries? A review of 273 baseball players with UCL injuries. J Shoulder Elbow Surg. 2014;23:1521–6.

30. Lee GA, Katz SD, Lazarus MN. Elbow valgus stress radiography in an uninjured population. Am J Sports Med. 1998;26:425–7.

31. Rijke AM, Goitz HT, McCue C, et al. Stress radiography of the medial elbow ligaments. Radiology. 1994;191:213–6.

32. Sasaki J, Takahara M, Ogino T, Kashiwa H, Ishigaki D, Kanauchi Y. Ultrasonographic assessment of the ulnar collateral ligament and medial elbow laxity in college baseball players. J Bone Joint Surg Am. 2002;84A(4):525–31.

33. Schwab GH, Bennett JB, Woods GW, Tullos HS. Biomechanics of elbow instability: the role of the medial collateral ligament. Clin Orthop. 1980;146:42–52.

34. Timmerman LA, Schwartz ML, Andrews JR. Preoperative evaluation of the ulnar collateral ligament by magnetic resonance imaging and computed tomography arthrography. Evaluation in 25 baseball players with surgical confirmation. Am J Sports Med. 1994;22:26–32.

35. Hill NB Jr, Bucchieri JS, Shon F, Miller TT, Rosenwasser MP. Magnetic resonance imaging of injury to the medial collateral ligament of the elbow: a cadaver model. J Shoulder Elbow Surg. 2000;9(5):418–22.

36. Munshi M, Pretterklieber ML, Chung CB, Haghighi P, Cho JH, Trudell DJ, et al. Anterior bundle of ulnar collateral ligament: evaluation of anatomic relationships by using MR imaging, MR arthrography, and gross anatomic and histologic analysis. Radiology. 2004;231(3):797–803.

37. Schwartz ML, Al-Zahrani S, Morwessel RM, et al. Ulnar collateral ligament injury in the throwing athlete: evaluation with saline-enhanced MR arthrography. Radiology. 1995;197:297–9.

38. Ahmad CS, Park KN, Elattrache KN. Elbow medial ulnar collateral ligament insufficiency alters posteromedial olecranon contact. Am J Sports Med. 2004;32(7):1607–12.

39. Rahman RK, Levine WN, Ahmad CS. Elbow medial collateral ligament injuries. Curr Rev Musculoskelet Med. 2008;1:197–204.

40. Ahmad CS, ElAttrache NS. Elbow valgus instability in the throwing athlete. J Am Acad Orthop Surg. 2006;14:693–700.

41. Rettig AC, Sherrill C, Snead DS, et al. Nonoperative treatment of ulnar collateral ligament injuries in throwing athletes. Am J Sports Med. 2001;29:15–7.

42. Kamineni S, ElAttrache NS, O'Driscoll SW, et al. Medial collateral ligament strain with partial posteromedial olecranon resection: biomechanical study. J Bone Joint Surg (Am). 2004;86:2424–30.

43. Conway JE, Jobe FW, Glousman RE, et al. Medial instability of the elbow in throwing athletes: treatment by repair or reconstruction of the ulnar collateral ligament. J Bone Joint Surg (Am). 1992;74:67–83.

44. Azar FM, Andrew JR, Wilk KE, et al. Operative treatment of ulnar collateral ligament injuries of the elbow in athletes. Am J Sports Med. 2000;28(1):16–23.

45. Eygendaal D, et al. Ligamentous reconstruction around the elbow using triceps tendon. Acta Orthop Scand. 2004;75(5):516–23.

46. Thompson WH, Jobe FW, Yocum LA, Pink MM. Ulnar collateral ligament reconstruction in athletes: muscle-splitting approach without transposition of the ulnar nerve. J Shoulder Elbow Surg. 2001;10:152–7.

47. Huh J, Krueger CA, Medvecky MJ, Hsu JR, et al. Medial Elbow exposure for coronoid fractures: FCU-split versus over-the-top. J Orthop Trauma. 2013;27:730–4.

48. Ahmad CS, Lee TQ, ElAttrache NS. Biomechanical evaluation of a new ulnar collateral ligament reconstruction technique with interference screw fixation. Am J Sports Med. 2003;31:332–7.

49. Rohrbough JT, Altchek DW, Hyman J, Williams RJ III, Botts JD. Medial collateral ligament reconstruction of the elbow using the docking technique. Am J Sports Med. 2002;30:541–8.

50. Jiang JJ, Leland JM. Analysis of pitching velocity in major league baseball players before and after ulnar collateral ligament reconstruction. Am J Sports Med. 2014;42:880–5.

51. Erickson BJ, Ak G, Harris JD, Bush-Joseph C, Bach BR, Abrams GD, San Juan AM, Cole BJ, Romeo AA. Rate of return to pitching and performance after Tommy John surgery in Major League Baseball pitchers. Am J Sports Med. 2014;42:536–43.

52. Jones KJ, Conte S, Patterson N, ElAttrache NS, Dines JS. Functional outcomes following revision ulnar collateral ligament reconstruction in Major League Baseball pitchers. J Shoulder Elbow Surg. 2013;22:642–6.

Posterolateral Rotatory Instability of the Elbow

Joideep Phadnis and Gregory I. Bain

5

Contents

J. Phadnis (✉)
Brighton & Sussex University Hospitals, Brighton &
Sussex Medical School, Brighton, UK
e-mail: joideep@doctors.org.uk

G. I. Bain
Department of Orthopaedic Surgery, Flinders
University and Flinders Medical Centre,
Adelaide, Australia
e-mail: greg@gregbain.com.au

© The Editor(s) (if applicable) and The Author(s), under exclusive license to Springer Nature
Switzerland AG 2021
A. C. Watts et al. (eds.), *Sports Injuries of the Elbow*, https://doi.org/10.1007/978-3-030-52379-4_5

Key Learning Points

1. PLRI is the most common form of elbow instability.
2. PLRI occurs because of injury to the LCLC of the elbow.
3. PLRI is caused by instability of the ulnohumeral joint—radial head dislocation is a consequence of this.
4. PLRI may be part of a more global form of elbow instability or part of a terrible triad injury.
5. The pivot shift test and posterolateral drawer test are commonly used to diagnose PLRI
6. Acute treatment consists of repair of the LCLC, while chronic PLRI requires reconstruction of the LCLC.
7. Bone loss contributing to PLRI must be addressed as part of the surgical treatment.
8. Outcomes after acute repair and chronic reconstruction are good.

5.1 Introduction

The term posterolateral rotatory instability (PLRI) of the elbow was coined by O'Driscoll in 1991 [1]. It refers to a syndrome of ulnohumeral instability, caused by injury to the lateral collateral ligament complex (LCLC), which results in posterior subluxation, or dislocation of the radial head relative to the capitellum. It is the most common form of elbow instability.

PLRI may be acute, chronic or iatrogenic and may occur purely as a result of soft tissue pathology or have a bony component.

Treatment of PLRI is determined by the cause and the other components of elbow instability that are present. Successful reparative or reconstructive surgery is dependent on recognising and treating each anatomic component that contributes to the instability pattern.

5.2 Pathoanatomy of PLRI

The elbow comprises three articulations: the ulnohumeral joint, the radiocapitellar joint and the proximal radioulnar joint. The ulnohumeral joint is highly congruent and inherently stable.

This articular congruency is the primary restraint of the elbow along with components of the lateral and medial collateral ligaments [2]. The secondary restraints are the radiocapitellar joint and the common flexor and common extensor muscles. A dynamic compressive force is also imparted by the Anconeus, Brachialis and Triceps muscles, which cross the joint [2, 3]. In particular the deep head of brachialis (anterior) and the anconeus (posterior) run either side of the radial head to provide a dynamic stabilising sling that protects the lateral collateral ligament during forced supination [4].

The essential lesion of PLRI is an injury to the lateral collateral ligament complex (LCLC). This was originally identified by Osborne and Cotterill [5] and has been refined by O'Driscoll and other authors [1, 6, 7].

The LCLC comprises of the radial collateral ligament (RCL), the lateral ulnar collateral ligament (LUCL), the annular ligament (AL) and the accessory collateral ligament (Fig. 5.1).

The RCL and LUCL share a common origin from the lateral epicondyle of the humerus, which is the isometric point for flexion and extension of the ulnohumeral joint [8]. The annular ligament is a layered structure that attaches posteriorly to the ulna in line with the supinator crest, blends anteriorly with the capsule of the ulnohumeral joint and attaches to the anterior lip of the lesser sigmoid notch of the ulna forming a capsule around the proximal radioulnar joint [9].

The RCL blends into the annular ligament, while the LUCL extends inferiorly and obliquely

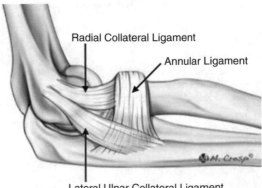

Radial Collateral Ligament

Annular Ligament

Lateral Ulnar Collateral Ligament

Fig. 5.1 Anatomy of the lateral collateral ligament complex

across the annular ligament to insert at the supinator crest of the ulna, immediately distal to the annular ligaments posterior insertion. This forms a hammock-like composite capsulo-ligamentous sheet, which captures the radial head [7, 9, 10]. The horizontal orientation of the RCL at the equator of the radial head is positioned to be the varus restraint of the ulnohumeral joint, whereas the oblique orientation of the LUCL, posterior to the equator of the radial head is positioned to be the primarily restraint to external rotation (supination) of the ulnohumeral joint. The LUCL is the only part of the LCLC that has a bony attachment to the humerus and ulna, and traditional teaching is that failure of the LUCL is the primary cause of PLRI [2, 7]. This has been disputed by biomechanical studies that suggest the whole LCLC needs to be disrupted before PLRI occurs [11–13] and by anatomic studies that found it difficult to consistently identify the individual components of the LCLC [13–15].

When the LCLC is injured it usually avulses from its humeral attachment as a sheet [1, 8, 16]. It translates distally to lie at the edge of the capitellar articular surface, where it is unable to heal [8]. The common extensor origin (CEO), which overlies the LCLC, may be intact with a concealed ligament injury beneath [2, 16]. Disruption of the CEO indicates a more severe injury to the elbow likely to result in a greater degree of instability [2, 8].

The most common bony form of PLRI is the terrible triad injury involving radial head fracture, coronoid fracture and elbow dislocation. By definition the LCLC is torn in this injury [2]. This failure occurs under tension as the ulnohumeral joint externally rotates. There are also frequently osteochondral lesions of the joint surfaces, particularly the capitellum, which may also have a posterior bone defect analogous to a Hill–Sachs lesion of the shoulder. In most cases, the coronoid fracture is a tip fracture located on the anterior or anterolateral aspect, sparring the MCL attachment on the anteromedial surface (sublime tubercle) [17]. The type of radial head fracture is determined by the position of the forearm and the degree of compression and shear imparted as the elbow dislocates. In severe injuries, there is also a rupture of the medial ligaments [8]. This sequen-

tial failure has been described as the Horii circle, where the injury propagates from lateral to medial across the elbow [2]. It has been suggested that, often, the medial structures remain intact with the elbow subluxating around the medial collateral ligament (MCL). Our experience has been that valgus instability persists after repair of the lateral structures. On exploration of the medial ligaments both components of the MCL are usually torn from their humeral attachment.

5.3 Mechanism of Injury

5.3.1 Traumatic

The classic mechanism of injury resulting in PLRI is a fall onto the outstretched hand, which imparts an axial, rotatory and valgus force on the elbow [8]. A valgus moment occurs because the mechanical axis of the body lies lateral to the elbow joint during a fall. The body rotates internally imparting an external rotation force on the elbow (supination), which is fixed by the planted hand [8]. This tensions the LCLC, which is ruptured from its humeral attachment. Consequently, the hammock containing the radial head is disrupted, leading to subluxation or dislocation of the radial head.

It is important to appreciate that the rotatory element of PLRI refers to ulnohumeral rotatory instability, and that radial head subluxation is a clinical marker of this instability, not the primary injury. In PLRI, the radial head subluxates because the proximal and distal radio-ulnar joints are intact, which means the ulna and radius rotate as a unit. This is distinct from an isolated radial head dislocation, where the proximal radioulnar joint is disrupted and the ulnohumeral joint remains intact [18].

5.3.2 Iatrogenic

PLRI may be caused by any iatrogenic injury to the LCLC. When performing lateral epicondylitis release, it is important to remain anterior to the equator of the radial head when elevating the extensor carpi radialis brevis from the lateral

Table 5.1 Aetiology of PLRI

	Pathoanatomy	Examples	Management
Traumatic	Soft tissue	Severe 'simple' dislocation	Consider acute soft tissue repair
	Bony	Fracture dislocation	Internal fixation and ligament repair
Atraumatic	Hyperlaxity	Ehlers-Danlos syndrome	Physio—if unhelpful then consider reconstruction with slow rehab (results inferior)
	Attenuation	Crutch walking	Orthotic modifications/reconstruction
		Inflammatory arthritis	Reconstruction/arthroplasty
		Varus humeral deformity	Corrective osteotomy and LCLC reconstruction
Iatrogenic	Surgical	Lateral/posterior surgical approaches	Reconstruction
		Radial head resection	Radial head replacement and LCLC reconstruction
	Medical	Multiple steroid injections or dry needling for tennis elbow	Reconstruction

epicondyle. Percutaneous release, dry needling or multiple steroid injections may compromise the collateral ligament.

The Kocher approach, through the interval between anconeus and extensor carpi ulnaris is a common surgical approach to the lateral elbow. By definition, a capsulotomy in the line of this approach will divide the LCLC. Consequently, we favour a 'Z' shaped capsulotomy, which facilitates an anatomic repair during closure [8]. Alternatively, a more anteriorly based approach, which spares the RCL and LUCL could be used [19].

Posterior approaches to the radiocapitellar joint, such as the Boyd approach or the Wrightington approach, require elevation of the LUCL and annular ligament from the supinator crest [19, 20]. These approaches should be avoided in the scenario of elbow instability where the LCLC is ruptured at the humerus, as they may cause a 'free floating' lateral collateral ligament.

5.3.3 Atraumatic

PLRI may result from chronic attenuation of the LCLC secondary to a chronic varus deformity of the distal humerus. Most commonly, this is due to a malunited supracondylar fracture during childhood. Cubitus varus results in asymmetric loading of the medial ulnohumeral joint and attenuation of the LCLC. This is exacerbated by triceps contraction, which lies medial to the axis of the elbow in cubitus varus

[21]. In this scenario, correction of the underlying deformity as well as reconstruction of the LCLC is necessary.

Chronic attenuation of the LCLC may also occur in a crutch-walking patient due to a cyclic posterolateral rotatory force. In these patients, modification to a forearm gutter may be enough to abate their symptoms and avoid the need for ligament reconstruction.

Patients with inflammatory arthritis may develop PLRI due to soft tissue attenuation and pannus formation. If suitable, linked arthroplasty may be considered in this group.

Finally, patients with global hyperlaxity or connective tissue disorders are more likely to develop PLRI without a history of trauma. The results of reconstructive surgery in this group are inferior and, hence, we are more conservative with rehabilitation if reconstructive surgery is performed [22, 23]. Table 5.1 summarises the aetiology of PLRI.

5.4 Clinical Presentation

5.4.1 History

Patients with PLRI may present acutely with an elbow dislocation, fracture dislocation or sub-acutely with symptoms of instability. These symptoms range from subtle to frank instability, however, it is more common for patients with isolated PLRI to only have subtle symptoms and signs. The patient may describe clunking, clicking or jarring, or they may just describe a feeling of apprehension. This is likely to be during provocative activities such as pushing up from a chair or doing press ups [24]. It can be very difficult for the patient to verbalise their sense of instability, hence any history of previous dislocation, lateral elbow surgery or generalised hyperlaxity should raise suspicion of PLRI.

5.4.2 Examination

All patients should be screened for generalised hyperlaxity and neurologic symptoms, particularly of the ulnar nerve. Inspection should identify previous surgical scars, especially on the lateral aspect and any abnormality to the carrying angle of the elbow. Generally, range of motion will be full and there may be hyperextension if there is no history of dislocation.

Both collateral ligaments should be tested. Although in pure PLRI only the lateral structures will be affected, the instability may be global and include the MCL. The MCL is stressed under valgus load in 15–30° flexion in order to unlock the ulnohumeral joint and relax the anterior capsule [24]. Some authors recommend testing the anterior bundle of the MCL in 60–90° [25, 26]. The forearm is pronated to tighten the radiocapitellar joint so that any excessive valgus will arise only from MCL deficiency. Varus testing in 30° flexion is performed to stress the LCLC, in particular the radial collateral ligament, however, in isolated PLRI there is usually no pure varus instability identified.

5.4.3 Provocation Tests

The two most common tests for PLRI are the pivot shift test (posterolateral rotatory instability test) and the posterolateral drawer test [1].

The pivot shift test is performed with the patient supine and the extremity over the patient's head. The shoulder is externally rotated, to stabilise the humerus, so that the elbow can be assessed independent of shoulder motion. The examiner grasps the patient's forearm, which is placed in full supination. Starting with supination and extension, the elbow is flexed while applying a valgus force and axial load. In this position, the ulna rotates externally on the trochlea subluxating the radial head posteriorly. At around 40°, the rotatory displacement is at a maximum and the subluxated radial head produces a skin dimple on the lateral aspect of the elbow. With further flexion, the triceps becomes taut and forces the radiocapitellar joint to reduce producing a "clunk" and change in the skin dimpling. Apprehension or pain, without a clunk during this manoeuvre should also be considered positive for PLRI.

In the posterolateral drawer test, the patient is positioned in the same way as for the pivot shift test. Anterior-posterior translation of the lateral forearm is performed whilst stabilising the humerus. The test is positive if a dimple appears on the lateral aspect of the elbow as the radial head subluxates then re-locates [24]. Apprehension should also be considered as a positive result.

Other provocative tests include asking the patient to push themselves up from a chair and to do a press up. Both actions impart a posterolateral rotatory force on the elbow and will reproduce the patients' symptoms [24].

All tests for PLRI may appear normal in the awake patient due to apprehension and guarding, however, joint proprioception may be dulled with an intra-articular local anaesthetic injection, which may unmask the underlying instability especially when examined under fluoroscopic control.

5.4.4 Imaging

Plain radiographs are useful to screen for deformity and osseous lesions, and may demonstrate a drop sign [27] (Fig. 5.2).

3D CT scans may reveal associated bony or chondral injuries indicative of instability, such as a coronoid tip fracture, radial head fracture or a capitellar Hill–Sachs lesion (Fig. 5.3). This reduces the range of radio-capitellar contact and

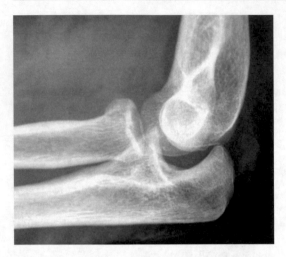

Fig. 5.2 X-ray demonstrating a drop sign. This is pathologic widening of the ulnohumeral joint without application of any stress. Note the incongruence of the ulnohumeral joint

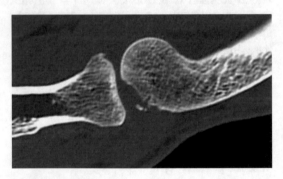

Fig. 5.3 Sagittal CT scan demonstrating a posterior impaction fracture of the capitellum also known as an Osborne Cotterill lesion. The lesion is usually not apparent on plain X-rays

predisposes to recurrent subluxation of the radial head [28].

MRI usually confirms rupture of the LCLC from the humeral insertion, although a normal appearing MRI should not rule out PLRI. MRI, is also valuable in identifying concurrent MCL injury and bone bruising or chondral damage to the coronoid, radial head or capitellum [29].

Dynamic fluoroscopy may ultimately be the only imaging modality to detect PLRI. Varus stress may not show gapping of the lateral joint line, however, a pivot shift test while viewing the elbow on a lateral view will show posterior subluxation of the radial head on the capitellum

or reveal the 'drop sign' [27]. This is pathologic widening of the ulnohumeral joint seen on the lateral view.

5.4.5 Arthroscopic Diagnosis

We routinely perform an arthroscopic assessment of these patients. We commence with dry arthroscopy, which yields a clearer image of the tissues and minimises distension of the joint, which may alter capsular laxity. Arthroscopy provides direct visual assessment of the bony, chondral and soft tissue stabilisers of the elbow, and allows dynamic instability testing.

Varus, valgus instability is assessed while viewing the anterior compartment looking for opening of the trochlea/coronoid interval during varus/valgus loading. A rent in the lateral capsule or detachment of the capsule from the lateral epicondyle may be seen.

Rotatory instability is assessed whilst viewing the posterior compartment. In PLRI, supination of the forearm may cause widening of the ulnohumeral articulation when viewing the lateral gutter (Fig. 5.4). In global instability there will also be widening of the medial ulnohumeral

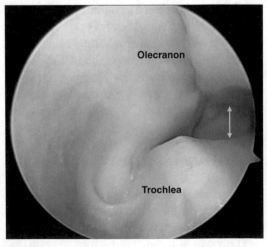

Fig. 5.4 Dry arthroscopy of a patient with PLRI. The lateral aspect of the ulnohumeral joint is viewed from the posterior compartment while supinating the forearm. Abnormal widening of the joint space (white arrow) is diagnostic of PLRI

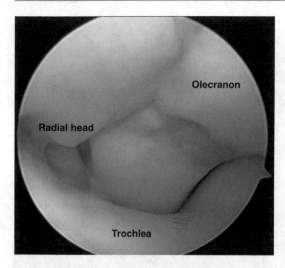

Fig. 5.5 Dry arthroscopy of a patient with global instability. A drive through sign is present where the arthroscope can be 'driven' into the anterior compartment from the posterior compartment because of instability

articulation with pronation (MCL rupture) and a drive through sign where the scope can be driven into the anterior compartment (Fig. 5.5).

5.5 Management

5.5.1 Acute Repair

In patients with a terrible triad injury to the elbow, a major component of surgical treatment is to primarily repair the LCLC. The elbow is approached through a global posterior approach or via a lateral incision [23]. Regardless of skin incision, the same deep approach is used. In severe cases the soft tissue injury will delineate the approach required, however, in many cases the CEO will be intact with a concealed LUCL injury beneath. The aim of LCLC repair is to recreate the sling effect of the LCLC around the radial head. Hence, we endeavour to maintain the posterolateral tissue as a single unit. Repair of the LCLC to the humerus can be performed using anchors, transosseous tunnels or a combination of the two [23, 30]. The aim is to restore the LCLC to its isometric point, at the centre of the capitellum. To achieve this we prefer to place anchors just proximal to the isometric point as

described by Moritomo et al. [31]. This reliably ensures restoration of the LCLC to its footprint at the isometric point. Care is taken to ensure the joint is reduced with the forearm pronated and the elbow in 45° flexion whilst tying the knots. If there is a more global instability we prefabricate the lateral repair without tying the sutures and then address the coronoid fracture, anterior capsule and/or MCL from the medial aspect. The sutures in each soft tissue component are then tied sequentially from lateral to medial.

Most 'simple' elbow dislocations do not require surgical stabilisation [32]. However, there is a subset of injuries that are grossly unstable that may need acute stabilisation. These injuries can be distinguished by the mechanism of injury (high energy or fall from height); the degree of swelling and bruising circumferentially around the elbow and by the patient's reluctance to mobilise their elbow after 1–2 weeks of non-operative treatment. We recommend examination under anaesthetic (EUA) of such patients and surgical stabilisation if the elbow dislocates during EUA. It is rare that such injuries have isolated PLRI, rather, they have a global instability pattern, the soft tissue component of which is far more dramatic than in a terrible triad injury. The whole distal humerus is often stripped of soft tissue and the joint is exposed as soon as a skin incision is made. Figure 5.6 illustrates EUA and then sequential ligament stabilisation of a grossly unstable 'simple' elbow dislocation.

5.5.2 Chronic Instability

The management of chronic PLRI is dependent on the patient's functional demands, the degree of instability and the pathoanatomy of the instability. Crutch walking patients or low demand patients with isolated PLRI that does not cause recurrent dislocation should be managed non-operatively if possible. However, most patients who present with chronic PLRI cannot be treated successfully with non-operative modalities such as bracing or physiotherapy.

If there is isolated LCLC insufficiency and only PLRI present we perform a LCLC reconstruction

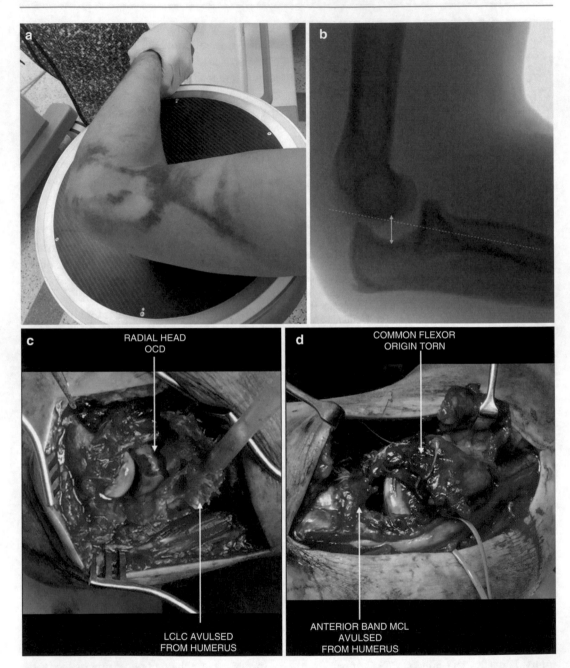

Fig. 5.6 Sequential stabilisation of a grossly unstable elbow with no bony injury (a 'simple' dislocation). (**a**) Examination under anaesthetic (EUA). Note the widespread bruising and swelling of the elbow. Valgus is applied with the weight of the forearm without excessive force by the surgeon. (**b**) EUA demonstrates widening of the ulnohumeral joint (arrow) and radiocapitellar malalignment (dotted line). Under only mild valgus load, the elbow is virtually dislocated. (**c**) Lateral incision and dissection through the superficial fascia. The LCLC has been avulsed from the lateral epicondyle with a significant tear of the common extensor origin. Note the osteochondral lesion of the radial head. (**d**) Medial incision reveals extensive underlying soft tissue damage down to the joint, without any further dissection. The MCL has been avulsed from its attachment on the humerus and the common flexor origin has been torn. (**e**) After repair of the LCLC, the radiocapitellar alignment has been restored (dotted line) but there is still ulnohumeral joint widening (arrow). (**f**) After repair of the MCL, the elbow is congruently reduced

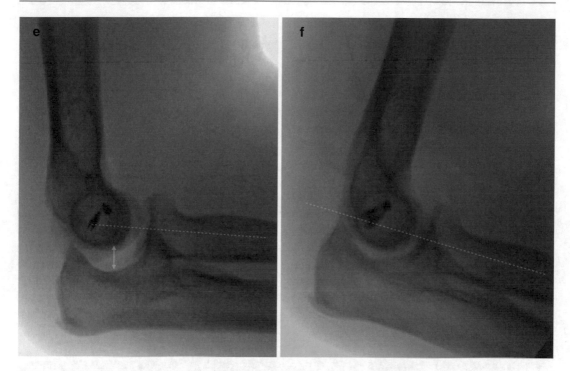

Fig. 5.6 (continued)

[23]. If there is combined PLRI and valgus insta-bility, then concurrent LCLC and MCL recon-struction is performed [33]. If there is also bony deficiency to the coronoid or radial head, these structures are also reconstructed [34].

5.5.3 Isolated LCLC Reconstruction

An autologous, isometric, extra-articular ten-don graft is our preference. Palmaris longus can be sufficient, however, it is often too small and hence hamstrings are preferred. On occasion we have used a flexor carpi radialis graft as this is in the same operative field and is much more robust than Palmaris longus. Other possible graft choices are allograft tendon, synthetic ligaments, triceps fascia or the fourth toe extensor tendon.

Whichever graft material and reconstruction technique is used, it is important to adequately tension the graft and to recreate the sling effect around the radial head.

5.5.4 Combined LCLC and MCL Reconstruction

If chronic valgus instability is present as well as PLRI it is important to address both components of the instability. This can be done by individu-ally reconstructing the LCLC and MCL or by performing a circumferential graft [22, 23]. The circumferential graft can be performed using a single or double loop technique [33]. The single loop technique is performed in all but the most complex cases.

5.5.5 Bone Loss

The primary osseous stabiliser of the ulnohu-meral joint is the coronoid process. Ulnohumeral instability is directly proportional to the amount of coronoid bone loss [17]. In chronic PLRI with coronoid bone loss it is generally not pos-sible to simply fix back the coronoid, as it may

have been fragmented or resorbed. In this scenario the coronoid process is reconstructed.
Autologous graft options include the radial
head, olecranon tip, rib and iliac crest. We prefer
not to use bone from the already unstable elbow
and feel that the iliac crest is inferior because it
lacks a cartilaginous surface. Hence we favour
using a costochondral graft harvested from the
sixth rib at the anterior costochondral junction
[34] (Fig. 5.7).

The radial head may contribute to instability
especially if it has been partially or completely
resected. The radial head, normally a secondary
stabiliser of the ulnohumeral joint, becomes of
prime importance when the MCL has been disrupted as it provides a restraint against valgus
stress [2]. Hence, it is prudent to fix or replace
the radial head to restore a congruent radiocapitellar articulation.

If present, posterior capitellar bone loss is not
usually reconstructed, as the primary pathology
of PLRI affects the ulnohumeral joint. The radiocapitellar instability seen on imaging and noted
on examination is a consequence of ulnohumeral
instability.

5.6   Outcomes

Several authors have reported good results after
both acute fixation and chronic reconstruction
of PLRI [22, 33, 35]. Recurrent instability is
uncommon, however patients with underlying
degenerative changes and hyperlaxity appear to
fare worse [18]. Reconstruction of PLRI after
cubitus varus and reconstruction after radial head
excision using radial head arthroplasty have been
reported with similarly good results [36, 37].

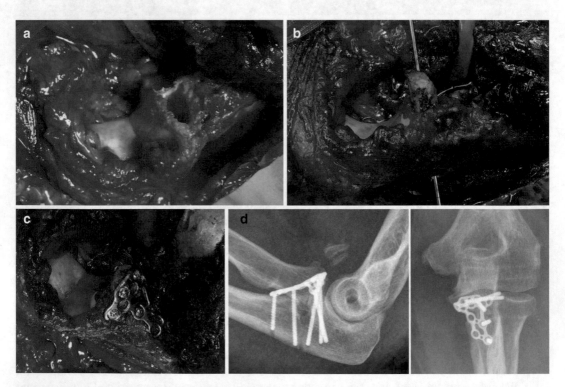

Fig. 5.7 A patient with chronic global instability and
coronoid bone loss, reconstructed with a costochondral
graft. (**a**) The native coronoid bed has been prepared to
allow insetting of the rib graft. (**b**) The rib graft has been
inset into the native coronoid bed and temporarily stabi-
lized with a Kirschner wire. (**c**) A buttress plate is applied
to ensure stability of the graft. (**d**) Post-operative X rays.
Note the fragmented native coronoid tip on the lateral
view and the humeral tunnel used to pass a circumferential graft

5.7   Conclusion

PLRI is a condition where failure of the LCLC results in ulnohumeral instability. PLRI should be considered as a part of a spectrum of elbow instability. Acute and chronic reconstruction should address all bony and soft tissue factors that contribute to PLRI. Doing so provides a good outcome in the majority of patients.

Q&A

Q1. What are the primary and secondary stabilisers of the elbow?

The primary stabilisers are the ulnohumeral joint, the lateral collateral ligament complex and the anterior band of the medial collateral ligament. The secondary stabilisers are the common flexor and extensor muscles groups, the radial head and the muscles that cross the elbow (brachialis, anconeus and triceps)

Q2. What are the components of the lateral collateral ligament complex?

These are the radial collateral ligament, the lateral ulna collateral ligament, the annular ligament and the accessory lateral collateral ligament

Q3. Why does the radial head dislocate in PLRI?

The radial head dislocates because the hammock effect of the LCLC is lost when it is ruptured. This means that when an external rotation force (supination) is applied to the elbow, the radial head is able to subluxate posterior to the capitellum.

Q4. What are the iatrogenic causes of PLRI?

Tennis elbow release performed posterior to the equator of the radial head. Surgical approaches (Kochers, Boyd and Wrightington approach) when not performed for the correct indication or without adequate repair. Previous radial head resection.

Q5. In chronic PLRI with bone loss, what options are there for coronoid reconstruction?

Autografts: Olecranon, radial head, iliac crest, costochondral.

Allografts may also be used although this is uncommon.

Q6. Which clinical tests are commonly used to diagnose PLRI?

The pivot shift test and the posterolateral drawer test are the two man provocative tests for PLRI. The armchair push up and press up tests are also useful provocative tests.

References

1. O'Driscoll SW, Bell DF, Morrey BF. Posterolateral rotatory instability of the elbow. J Bone Joint Surg Am. 1991;73(3):440–6.
2. O'Driscoll SW, Jupiter JB, King GJ, Hotchkiss RN, Morrey BF. The unstable elbow. J Bone Joint Surg Am. 2000;82(5):724–38.
3. Mehta JA, Bain GI. Elbow dislocations in adults and children. Clin Sports Med. 2004;23(4):609–27.
4. Leonello DT, Galley IJ, Bain GI, Carter CD. Brachialis muscle anatomy. A study in cadavers. J Bone Joint Surg Am. 2007;89(6):1293-7.
5. Osborne G, Cotterill P. Recurrent dislocation of the elbow. J Bone Joint Surg Br. 1966;48(2):340–6. British Editorial Society of Bone and Joint Surgery.
6. McAdams TR, Masters GW, Srivastava S. The effect of arthroscopic sectioning of the lateral ligament complex of the elbow on posterolateral rotatory stability. J Shoulder Elb Surg. 2005;14(3):298–301.
7. Morrey BF, An KN. Functional anatomy of the ligaments of the elbow. Clin Orthop Relat Res. 1985;201:84–90.
8. Mehta JA, Bain GI. Posterolateral rotatory instability of the elbow. J Am Acad Orthop Surg. 2004;12:405–15.
9. Martin BF. The annular ligament of the superior radio-ulnar joint. J Anat. 1958;92(Pt 3):473.
10. Seki A, Olsen BS, Jensen SL, Eygendaal D, Søjbjerg JO. Functional anatomy of the lateral collateral ligament complex of the elbow: configuration of Y and its role. J Shoulder Elb Surg. 2002;11(1):53–9.
11. Dunning CE, Zarzour ZD, Patterson SD, Johnson JA, King GJ. Ligamentous stabilizers against posterolateral rotatory instability of the elbow. J Bone Joint Surg Am. 2001;83-A(12):1823–8.
12. Olsen BS, Søjbjerg JO, Dalstra M, Sneppen O. Kinematics of the lateral ligamentous constraints of the elbow joint. J Shoulder Elb Surg. 1996;5(5):333–41.
13. Olsen BS, Vaesel MT, Søjbjerg JO, Helmig P, Sneppen O. Lateral collateral ligament of the elbow joint: anatomy and kinematics. J Shoulder Elb Surg. 1996;5(2 Pt 1):103–12.

14. Cohen MS, Hastings H II. Rotatory instability of the elbow. The anatomy and role of the lateral stabilizer. J Bone Joint Surg Am. 1997;79(2):225–33.

15. Imatani J, Ogura T, Morito Y, Hashizume H, Inoue H. Anatomic and histologic studies of lateral collateral ligament complex of the elbow joint. J Shoulder Elb Surg. 1999;8(6):625–7.

16. McKee MD, Schemitsch EH, Sala MJ, O'Driscoll SW. The pathoanatomy of lateral ligamentous disruption in complex elbow instability. J Shoulder Elb Surg. 2003;12(4):391–6.

17. Doornberg JN, Ring D. Coronoid fracture patterns. YJHSU. 2006;31(1):45–52.

18. Charalambous CP, Stanley JK. Posterolateral rotatory instability of the elbow. J Bone Joint Surg. 2008;90(3):272–9. British Volume. British Editorial Society of Bone and Joint Surgery.

19. Cheung EV, Steinmann SP. Surgical approaches to the elbow. J Am Acad Orthop Surg. 2009;17:325–33.

20. Stanley JK, Penn DS, Wasseem M. Exposure of the head of the radius using the Wrightington approach. J Bone Joint Surg (Br). 2006;88(9):1178–82.

21. Beuerlein MJ, Reid JT, Schemitsch EH, McKee MD. Effect of distal humeral varus deformity on strain in the lateral ulnar collateral ligament and ulnohumeral joint stability. J Bone Joint Surg Am. 2004;86-A(10):2235–42.

22. Finkbone PR, O'Driscoll SW. Box-loop ligament reconstruction of the elbow for medial and lateral instability. J Shoulder Elb Surg. 2015;24(4):647–54.

23. McGuire D, Bain GI. Medial and lateral collateral ligament repair or reconstruction of the elbow. Oper Tech Orthop. 2013;23(4):205–14.

24. Morrey BF, Sanchez-Sotelo J. The elbow and its disorders. 4th ed: Elsevier Health Sciences; 2009.

25. Hariri S, Safran MR. Ulnar collateral ligament injury in the overhead athlete. Clin Sports Med. 2010;29(4):619–44.

26. O'Driscoll SW, Lawton RL, Smith AM. The "moving valgus stress test" for medial collateral ligament tears of the elbow. Am J Sports Med. Am Orthopaed Soc Sports Med. 2005;33(2):231–9.

27. Coonrad RW, Roush TF, Major NM, Basamania CJ. The drop sign, a radiographic warning sign of elbow instability. J Shoulder Elb Surg. 2005;14(3):312–7.

28. Shukla DR, Thoreson AR, Fitzsimmons JS, An K-N, O'Driscoll SW. The effect of capitellar impaction fractures on radiocapitellar stability. J Hand Surg. 2015;40(3):520–5.

29. Sampath SC, Sampath SC, Bredella MA. Magnetic resonance imaging of the elbow: a structured approach. Sports Health. 2013;5(1):34–49.

30. Lee YC, Eng K, Keogh A, McLean JM, Bain GI. Repair of the acutely unstable elbow: use of tensionable anchors. Tech Hand Up Extrem Surg. 2012;16(4):225–9.

31. Moritomo H, Murase T, Arimitsu S, Oka K, Yoshikawa H, Sugamoto K. The in vivo isometric point of the lateral ligament of the elbow. J Bone Joint Surg Am. 2007;89(9):2011–7.

32. Josefsson PO, Gentz CF, Johnell O, Wendeberg B. Surgical versus non-surgical treatment of ligamentous injuries following dislocation of the elbow joint. A prospective randomized study. J Bone Joint Surg Am. 1987;69(4):605–8.

33. van Riet RP, Bain GI, Baird R, Lim YW. Simultaneous reconstruction of medial and lateral elbow ligaments for instability using a circumferential graft. Tech Hand Up Extrem Surg. 2006;10(4):239–44.

34. Silveira GH, Bain GI, Eng K. Reconstruction of coronoid process using costochondral graft in a case of chronic posteromedial rotatory instability of the elbow. J Shoulder Elbow Surg. 2013;22(5):e14–8.

35. Sanchez-Sotelo J, Morrey BF, O'Driscoll SW. Ligamentous repair and reconstruction for posterolateral rotatory instability of the elbow. J Bone Joint Surg (Br). 2005;87(1):54–61.

36. Hall JA, McKee MD. Posterolateral rotatory instability of the elbow following radial head resection. J Bone Joint Surg Am. 2005;87(7):1571–9.

37. O'Driscoll SW, Spinner RJ, McKee MD, Kibler WB, Hastings H, Morrey BF, et al. Tardy posterolateral rotatory instability of the elbow due to cubitus varus. J Bone Joint Surg Am. 2001;83-A(9):1358–69.

Osteochondritis Dissecans of the Elbow

6

Christiaan J. A. van Bergen, Kimberly I. M. van den Ende, and Denise Eygendaal

Contents

Key Learning Points

Osteochondritis dissecans of the elbow:

1. is a lesion of the articular cartilage and subchondral bone that typically affects the capitellum of the humerus

2. usually presents in young athletes engaged in repetitive overhead or upper extremity weight-bearing activities

3. should be suspected in any teenager presenting with lateral elbow pain, since delay in the diagnosis is common

4. is diagnosed with use of computed tomography or magnetic resonance imaging

5. is initially treated nonoperatively if stable (characterised by an open growth plate and flattening or radiolucency of the subchondral bone in a patient with normal elbow motion)

C. J. A. van Bergen (✉) · K. I. M. van den Ende
D. Eygendaal
Department of Orthopaedic Surgery, Amphia Hospital, Breda, The Netherlands
e-mail: cvanbergen@amphia.nl;
deygendaal@amphia.nl

A. C. Watts et al. (eds.), *Sports Injuries of the Elbow*, https://doi.org/10.1007/978-3-030-52379-4_6

6. is treated surgically if refractory to nonoperative treatment or if unstable

6.1 Introduction

Osteochondritis dissecans (OCD) is a process in which a segment of articular cartilage separates from the subchondral bone. In the human body, OCD lesions are most commonly found in the knee, followed by the ankle and the elbow [1]. OCD of the elbow typically affects the capitellum of the humerus. It can be a debilitating injury in a young patient population.

6.1.1 Epidemiology

Elbow OCD presents typically in adolescent athletes engaged in repetitive overhead or upper extremity weight-bearing activities (e.g. baseball, tennis, volleyball, weight lifting and gymnastics). The prevalence of OCD of the humeral capitellum was 3.4% among more than 2000 adolescent baseball players [2]. Not all of these patients had symptoms [2]. Patients with an OCD usually are in their second decade of life, with an age ranging from 11 to 23 years. Boys are affected more commonly than girls. The capitellum of the dominant elbow is mostly affected. Bilateral involvement is seen in up to 20% of the patients [3].

Elbow OCD should be distinguished from Panner's disease or osteochondrosis of the capitellum. Panner's disease is encountered in younger children (aged 4–12 years), and characterised by ischaemia and necrosis of the capitellar epiphysis, followed by regeneration and recalcification. It is a self-limiting, benign disorder that usually resolves with rest.

6.1.2 Aetiology

The exact aetiology of OCD is unknown. A genetic predisposition has been suggested in twin studies [4]. The main cause, however, is thought to be excessive repetitive valgus compression across the elbow joint with immature articular cartilage [5, 6]. Repetitive stress to the lateral elbow compartment could lead to localised injury

of subchondral bone of the poorly vascularised humeral capitellum, characterised by focal avascular necrosis and subchondral bone changes. Subsequently, this could result in loss of support for the overlying articular cartilage and eventually breakdown and formation of loose fragments once the mechanical support of the articular cartilage is compromised [5, 6].

6.1.3 Pathology

OCD usually evolves through three stages [3, 6]. In stage 1, hyperemic bone and oedematous periarticular soft tissues are found. In stage 2, the epiphysis deforms, sometimes with fragmentation. In stage 3, necrotic bone is replaced by granulation tissue. The articular surface may separate and form a loose body as the bone heals.

6.1.4 Natural History

It seems logical to assume that patients with OCD are predisposed to early osteoarthritis of the elbow. However, the relation between cartilage defects in general and the development of osteoarthritis in the long term has not been elucidated to date. Most evidence is available for cartilage lesions in the knee and ankle [7, 8]. Large chondral and osteochondral lesions of the knee are presumed to predispose to osteoarthritis, although the scientific evidence is limited [7]. In the ankle, however, a relation between OCD and osteoarthritis has not been shown [8]. Only 4% of ankle OCDs develop a narrowed joint space up to 20 years of follow-up [9].

With regard to the elbow, little is known about the risk of developing degenerative changes in the long term. Bauer et al. [10] investigated elbow degeneration amongst 31 OCD patients at a mean follow-up of 23 years. One-third had radiographic degenerative changes and 42% of patients complained of pain and/or reduced range of motion at the time of follow-up. Younger patients had better odds of having a pain-free elbow without radiographic signs of degeneration in the long term. In addition, larger lesions may be more prone to degenerative changes over time. Takahara et al. [11] noted a poorer long-term outcome of patients with large cartilage lesions compared with those with small lesions. There is no evidence that surgical debridement with or without microfracturing protects against degeneration.

6.2 Clinical Presentation

Patient's delay and doctor's delay are very common in elbow OCD. Therefore, a high index of suspicion and directed imaging studies are necessary. In fact, any teenager presenting with lateral elbow pain should be suspected of having an OCD lesion. The typical patient is a young male sports person, initially presenting with pain, tenderness, and swelling over the lateral aspect of the elbow [12]. In a later stage, there may be loss of extension and intermittent catching and locking of the elbow, but physical examination findings are not very distinct in the early stage of OCD. Yet, it is important to detect OCD as early as possible to prevent expansion of the lesion and possible degeneration of the joint.

6.3 Imaging

Plain anteroposterior and lateral radiographs are often used as an initial screening method (Fig. 6.1). Radiographic signs of an OCD are flattening of the capitellum, a focal defect of the articular surface, and loose bodies. However, routine radiographs of the elbow are insensitive in identifying OCD of the capitellum [13]. In fact, approximately half of the radiographs of patients with a capitellar OCD appear normal [13]. An anteroposterior view with the elbow in 45° of flexion may better depict the lesion [14].

Because of the low sensitivity of plain radiography, additional imaging is indicated when an OCD is suspected. Ultrasound of the elbow has been described to detect capitellar OCD [15–17]. However, the capitellum is partially obscured by the radial head [17]. Computed tomography (CT) and magnetic resonance imaging (MRI) are most useful in diagnosing an OCD. MRI demonstrates early OCD and is valuable in determining the stability and viability of the OCD fragment (Fig. 6.2) [10, 17, 18].

CT scans, however, are more sensitive and better depict loose bodies (Fig. 6.3). We studied 25 patients with an OCD proven by arthroscopy who all had preoperative radiographs, MRI and CT [19]. The OCD was visible on 25 CT scans (sensitivity, 100%), on 24 MRI scans (sensitivity, 96%), and on 19 radiographs (sensitivity, 76%). Arthroscopy identified loose bodies in 20 cases. These were visible in 18 CT scans (90%), 13 MRI scans (65%) and 11 radiographs (55%). CT thus seems to be the best imaging technique to diagnose OCD and loose bodies.

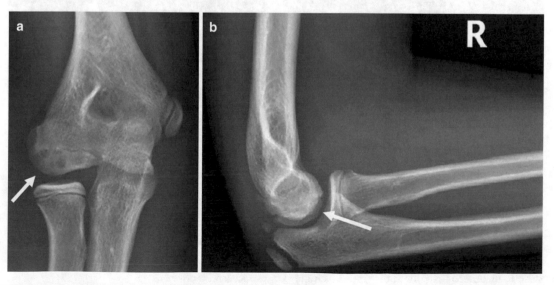

Fig. 6.1 Plain radiography of the elbow (**a**, anteroposterior; **b**, lateral) showing an osteochondritis dissecans lesion of the capitellum

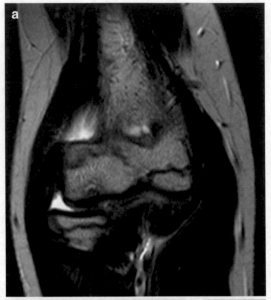

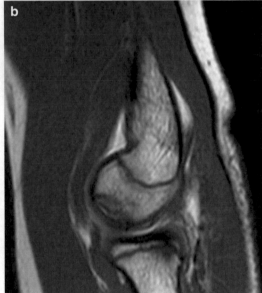

Fig. 6.2 Magnetic resonance imaging (**a**, coronal view; **b**, sagittal view) of an elbow affected with osteochondritis dissecans of the capitellum

6.3.1 Classification

Although the value of grading capitellar OCD seems limited, various classifications have been described. Most are based on radiography, MRI, or arthroscopy.

Minami et al. [20] described a classification based on anteroposterior radiography. Grade 1

describes a stable lesion with a translucent cystic shadow in the capitellum; grade 2, a clear zone between the OCD and adjacent subchondral bone; and grade 3, loose bodies.

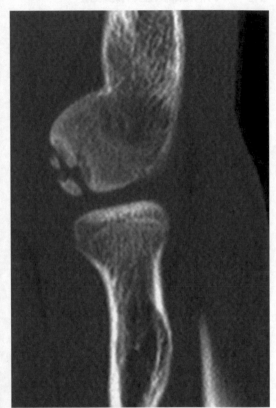

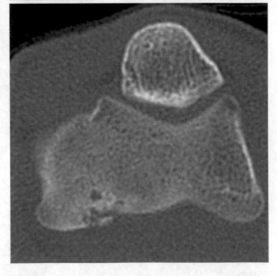

Fig. 6.3 Computed tomography scans showing capitellar osteochondritis dissecans

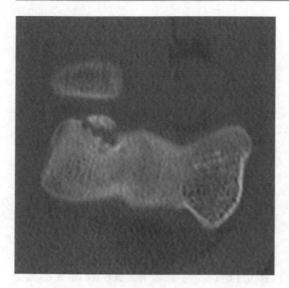

Fig. 6.3 (continued)

Itsubo et al. [21] recently introduced a T2-weighted MRI staging system that provides accurate and reliable estimation of stability of OCD. The following stages are distinguished: stage 1, normally shaped capitellum with several spotted areas of high signal intensity that is lower than that of cartilage; stage 2, as with stage 1 but with several spotted areas of higher intensity than that of cartilage; stage 3, as with stage 2 but with both discontinuity and noncircularity of the chondral surface signal of the capitellum and no high signal interface apparent between the lesion and the floor; stage 4, lesion separated by a high intensity line in comparison with cartilage; and stage 5, capitellar lesion displaced from the floor or defect of the capitellar lesion noted. Stages 1 and 2 are considered stable. Stages 3, 4 and 5 are considered unstable.

The International Cartilage Repair Society has proposed an arthroscopic classification system for OCD lesions [22]. Grade 1 indicates a stable lesion with a continuous but softened area covered by intact cartilage; grade 2, a lesion with partial discontinuity that is stable when probed; grade 3, a lesion with a complete discontinuity that is not yet dislocated; and grade 4, an empty defect as well as a defect with a dislocated fragment or a loose fragment lying within the bed.

6.4 Treatment and Outcomes

The treatment choice depends on several aspects, including the severity of symptoms and the size, location and stability of the lesion. It is important to differentiate between stable and unstable OCD lesions. In general, stable lesions may be reversible and can heal completely with nonoperative management, while unstable lesions need surgical treatment [23]. Stable lesions are characterised by an immature capitellum with an open growth plate, and flattening or radiolucency of the subchondral bone, in a patient with (almost) normal elbow motion [23, 24]. Unstable lesions have at least one of the following findings: a capitellum with a closed growth plate, fragmentation, or restriction of elbow motion 20° or more [23, 25]. On MRI, unstable lesions are characterised by a high signal intensity line through the articular cartilage, a high signal intensity interface, and an articular defect [13, 21].

6.4.1 Nonoperative Treatment

Nonoperative measures consist of rest or sports restriction (cessation of repetitive stress on the elbow), muscle strengthening exercises, non-steroidal anti-inflammatory drugs, and/or a short course of immobilisation [23, 24, 26]. The minority of OCD lesions are classified as stable and the initial success rates of nonoperative treatment were poor [23, 27]. Takahara et al. [27] reported a success rate of only 50% after an average follow-up of 12.6 years. Factors that are associated with the outcomes of nonoperative treatment were identified later. Bradley and Petrie [26] reported that most patients fully recovered with complete return to sports with rest alone if they had a lesion with all of the following conditions: 1, open capitellar growth plate; 2, localised flattening or radiolucency of the subchondral bone; and 3, good elbow motion. Likewise, Mihara et al. [24] showed that spontaneous healing potential of OCD in patients with open capitellar growth plates appears high. Conversely, healing potential with nonoperative management is extremely low in advanced OCD lesions with closed growth plates and in those that are unstable, even if they are undisplaced [6, 10, 24, 26, 27].

6.4.2 Surgical Treatment

Although outcome studies on surgical treatment lack long-term follow-up and have limited methodologic quality, they generally show satisfactory results regarding pain, return to sports, and elbow function [28]. Surgical intervention is, therefore, indicated for lesions that do not respond to initial nonoperative treatment and for unstable lesions [28].

Primary surgical management most commonly consists of arthroscopic debridement of the lesion, microfracturing of the subchondral bone and removal of loose fragments. Alternatively, to arthroscopic surgery or for lesions after failed previous surgery, numerous open surgical approaches have been reported, including internal fixation of large fragments and osteochondral autograft transfer [14, 29–32].

6.4.2.1 Arthroscopic Treatment

Arthroscopic surgery has become the standard procedure for the treatment of capitellar OCD [33]. It offers the advantage of direct visualisation of the pathology and the ability to treat the lesion through small stab incisions. This minimally invasive approach reduces the risk of operative morbidity and allows the patient to start rehabilitation directly after surgery [33].

Arthroscopic treatment consists of debridement of the lesion to achieve a stable rim, followed by bone marrow stimulation, and removal of any loose fragments and osteophytes [34, 35]. The patient is placed in the lateral decubitus position on the operating table. A tourniquet is placed around the upper arm, which rests on a padded arm holder that is attached to the side of the table (Fig. 6.4).

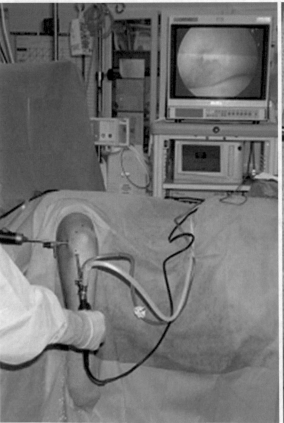
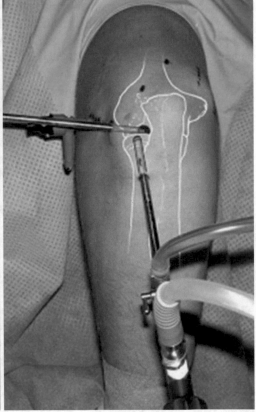

Fig. 6.4 Patient positioning for arthroscopy of a left elbow. The patient is in the lateral decubitus position and the arm rests on a support

The portal sites and the ulnar nerve are marked, and the elbow is disinfected and draped. The joint is injected with 20 mL of saline solution. The complete elbow joint is inspected from anterior and posterior with use of five to six portals. A distal ulnar portal allows for ergonomic exposure to the posterolateral capitellum providing easy access for drilling, burring and local debridement [33]. A bonecutter shaver or curette is brought into the posterolateral capitellar joint space through the standard soft-spot lateral portal. All unstable cartilage and necrotic bone are removed. Any cysts underlying the defect are opened and curetted. After debridement, several connections with the subchondral bone are created by drilling with a Kirschner wire or microfracturing with an awl (Fig. 6.5).

The objective is to partially destroy the calcified zone that is often present and to create openings into the subchondral bone. Intraosseous blood vessels are disrupted and the release of growth factors leads to the formation of a fibrin clot. The formation of local new blood vessels is stimulated, marrow cells are introduced in the defect, and fibrocartilaginous tissue is formed [36, 37].

Arthroscopic treatment has shown encouraging results at intermediate follow-up [34, 35, 37, 38]. Most studies report significant improvement in clinical outcome scores up to 9 years of follow-up [34, 35, 37–39]. Approximately 80–90% of patients return to sports and time to return to sports varies from 1 month to 5 months [40–42]. Complications of elbow arthroscopy are seen in 7–14% of cases [43, 44]. Most complications are minor, e.g. superficial wound problems and transient nerve palsies not affecting clinical outcome. Major complications occur in 0.5–5% of cases (e.g. deep infection, permanent nerve injury, or complications requiring additional anaesthesia) [43, 44].

6.4.2.2 Open Surgical Treatment

Refixation of the lesion can be indicated for large and (sub)acute osteochondral fragments [30, 31, 45]. Different fixation techniques are available, including metal and bioresorbable screws [30], pull-out wiring [31, 46], and corticocancellous bone pegs from the iliac crest or olecranon process [3]. Cancellous bone can be additionally grafted into the defect to enhance union of the fragment [30, 31].

In follow-up studies, the clinical success rate of refixation is approximately 80% [45–47]. Reossification is observed in 44–100% at follow-up [30, 31, 46]. An intact lateral wall of the capitellum appears to be important for fixation to be successful [47]. Complications have been observed in terms of intra-articular protrusion and loosening of screws [26].

After successful application in the knee and ankle [48], autologous osteochondral transplantation (or mosaicplasty) has been used in repairing OCD lesions of the humeral capitellum. With this technique, cylindrical osteochondral grafts are harvested from a non-weight-bearing area at the proximal aspect of the lateral femoral condyle and transplanted to the elbow to resurface the capitellar OCD.

Several authors have evaluated the technique [29, 32, 49, 50]. In a series of ten patients, eight were completely pain free after a mean follow-up of 30 months [50]. In a recent investigation of 33 patients who were allowed to begin throwing after 3 months and to return to sports after 6 months, 31 patients returned to a competitive level at which they had previously played after a mean of 7 months [49]. Although the clinical

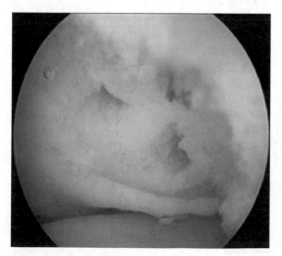

Fig. 6.5 Arthroscopic picture showing an osteochondritis dissecans lesion after debridement and microfracturing

outcomes are encouraging, the grafting technique implies damaging a healthy knee joint, possibly leading to donor-site morbidity. In a study that addressed the effect of the harvesting on donor knee function in young athletes, a time lag was evident in recovery between postoperative symptoms and muscle power at 3 months [51]. However, harvesting osteochondral grafts did not exert adverse effects at 2 years after the procedure [51].

Osteochondral autograft transfer has the advantage of replacing the affected articular surface with hyaline cartilage, but it is an invasive procedure with possible donor-site morbidity. Therefore, we recommend reserving this method for revision cases after failed primary arthroscopic treatment.

Other open procedures in the literature include rib osteochondral autograft and capitellar correction osteotomy [52–54]. Rib autografting provided satisfactory results after a follow-up of 1–6 years for advanced OCD with extensive lesions ≥15 mm and those affecting the lateral wall [53, 54]. Closed-wedge osteotomy of the capitellum has been described to widen the radiohumeral joint space, reduce compression, and stimulate revascularization and remodelling of the area of the lesion in the capitellum [52]. Although almost all patients returned to full athletic activity, postoperative osteoarthritic changes and enlargement of the radial head occurred in all patients. Because of the few scientific data, the place of these experimental treatment methods is unclear until more evidence is available.

6.4.3 Postoperative Rehabilitation

A physical therapist supervises the rehabilitation after surgery. Rehabilitation is aimed at reducing pain and swelling and restoring range of motion. The recovery after arthroscopic treatment is usually faster than after open surgery [3]. Active-assisted motion exercises are started within a couple of days after surgery. After arthroscopy, the range of motion is unrestricted as pain toler-

ates. For patients who were treated by mosaicplasty, flexion is restricted for the first 6 weeks. Resistive exercises are begun at 8 weeks after arthroscopic treatment and at 12 weeks after open treatment. If the patient has no pain and normal range of motion, an interval throwing program is initiated before the patient returns to sports [3].

6.5 Conclusions

OCD of the elbow typically affects the humeral capitellum of adolescent throwing athletes and leads to pain on the lateral aspect of the joint. CT or MRI are indicated to confirm the diagnosis and to address stability of the lesion. Nonoperative treatment can be initiated for stable lesions. Arthroscopic surgery has become the standard primary surgical procedure for treatment of capitellar OCD. This minimally invasive approach shows good results, low risk of operative morbidity, and early recuperation postoperatively. Open surgery is indicated for more advanced cases or for those that failed previous operative treatment.

Q&A
Q: Which part of the elbow is mostly affected by OCD?
A: The capitellum of the humerus
Q: What kind of patient usually presents with OCD?
A: An adolescent athlete engaged in repetitive overhead or upper extremity weight-bearing activities
Q: What is the best imaging study to diagnose OCD and loose bodies?
A: Computed tomography
Q: What is the primary surgical treatment?
A: Arthroscopic debridement and bone marrow stimulation
Q: Which open surgical procedure are available?
A: Fragment fixation, knee osteochondral autograft transfer (mosaicplasty), rib osteochondral autograft, and capitellar correction osteotomy

References

1. Bruns J. Osteochondrosis dissecans. Orthopade. 1997;26(6):573–84.
2. Kida Y, Morihara T, Kotoura Y, Hojo T, Tachiiri H, Sukenari T, et al. Prevalence and clinical characteristics of osteochondritis dissecans of the humeral capitellum among adolescent baseball players. Am J Sports Med. 2014;42(8):1963–71.
3. Baratz M, Yi SJ. Osteochondritis dissecans of the elbow. In: Eygendaal D, editor. The elbow. The treatment of basic elbow pathology. Nieuwegein: Arko Sports Media; 2009. p. 139–48.
4. Kenniston JA, Beredjiklian PK, Bozentka DJ. Osteochondritis dissecans of the capitellum in fraternal twins: case report. J Hand Surg Am. 2008;33(8):1380–3.
5. Douglas G, Rang M. The role of trauma in the pathogenesis of the osteochondroses. Clin Orthop Relat Res. 1981;158:28–32.
6. Takahara M, Ogino T, Takagi M, Tsuchida H, Orui H, Nambu T. Natural progression of osteochondritis dissecans of the humeral capitellum: initial observations. Radiology. 2000;216(1):207–12.
7. Heijink A, Gomoll AH, Madry H, Drobnic M, Filardo G, Espregueira-Mendes J, et al. Biomechanical considerations in the pathogenesis of osteoarthritis of the knee. Knee Surg Sports Traumatol Arthrosc. 2012;20(3):423–35.
8. Van Dijk CN, Reilingh ML, Zengerink M, van Bergen CJ. The natural history of osteochondral lesions in the ankle. Instr Course Lect. 2010;59:375–86.
9. van Bergen CJ, Kox LS, Maas M, Sierevelt IN, Kerkhoffs GM, van Dijk CN. Arthroscopic treatment of osteochondral defects of the talus: outcomes at eight to twenty years of follow-up. J Bone Joint Surg Am. 2013;95(6):519–25.
10. Bauer M, Jonsson K, Josefsson PO, Linden B. Osteochondritis dissecans of the elbow. A long-term follow-up study. Clin Orthop Relat Res. 1992;284:156–60.
11. Takahara M, Ogino T, Sasaki I, Kato H, Minami A, Kaneda K. Long term outcome of osteochondritis dissecans of the humeral capitellum. Clin Orthop Relat Res. 1999;363:108–15.
12. Takahara M, Shundo M, Kondo M, Suzuki K, Nambu T, Ogino T. Early detection of osteochondritis dissecans of the capitellum in young baseball players. Report of three cases. J Bone Joint Surg Am. 1998;80(6):892–7.
13. Kijowski R, De Smet AA. Radiography of the elbow for evaluation of patients with osteochondritis dissecans of the capitellum. Skeletal Radiol. 2005;34(5):266–71.
14. Takahara M, Mura N, Sasaki J, Harada M, Ogino T. Classification, treatment, and outcome of osteochondritis dissecans of the humeral capitellum. Surgical technique. J Bone Joint Surg Am. 2008;90(Suppl 2 Pt):147–62.
15. Harada M, Takahara M, Sasaki J, Mura N, Ito T, Ogino T. Using sonography for the early detection of elbow injuries among young baseball players. AJR Am J Roentgenol. 2006;187(6):1436–41.
16. Takahara M, Ogino T, Tsuchida H, Takagi M, Kashiwa H, Nambu T. Sonographic assessment of osteochondritis dissecans of the humeral capitellum. AJR Am J Roentgenol. 2000;174(2):411–5.
17. Takenaga T, Goto H, Nozaki M, Yoshida M, Nishiyama T, Otsuka T. Ultrasound imaging of the humeral capitellum: a cadaveric study. J Orthop Sci. 2014;19(6):907–12.
18. Dewan AK, Chhabra AB, Khanna AJ, Anderson MW, Brunton LM. MRI of the elbow: techniques and spectrum of disease: AAOS exhibit selection. J Bone Joint Surg Am. 2013;95(14):e99-13.
19. van den Ende KIM, Keijsers R, van den Bekerom MPJ, Eygendaal D. Imaging and classification of osteochondritis dissecans of the capitellum: X-ray, magnetic resonance imaging or computed tomography? Shoulder Elb. 2019;11(2):129–36. https://doi.org/10.1177/1758573218756866.
20. Minami M, Nakashita K, Ishii S, Usui M, Muramatsu I. Twenty-five cases of osteochondritis dissecans of the elbow. Rinsho Seikei Geka. 1979:14805–10.
21. Itsubo T, Murakami N, Uemura K, Nakamura K, Hayashi M, Uchiyama S, et al. Magnetic resonance imaging staging to evaluate the stability of capitellar osteochondritis dissecans lesions. Am J Sports Med. 2014;42(8):1972–7.
22. Brittberg M, Winalski CS. Evaluation of cartilage injuries and repair. J Bone Joint Surg Am. 2003;85(Suppl):258–69.
23. Takahara M, Mura N, Sasaki J, Harada M, Ogino T. Classification, treatment, and outcome of osteochondritis dissecans of the humeral capitellum. J Bone Joint Surg Am. 2007;89(6):1205–14.
24. Mihara K, Tsutsui H, Nishinaka N, Yamaguchi K. Nonoperative treatment for osteochondritis dissecans of the capitellum. Am J Sports Med. 2009;37(2):298–304.
25. Satake H, Takahara M, Harada M, Maruyama M. Preoperative imaging criteria for unstable osteochondritis dissecans of the capitellum. Clin Orthop Relat Res. 2013;471(4):1137–43.
26. Bradley JP, Petrie RS. Osteochondritis dissecans of the humeral capitellum. Diagnosis and treatment. Clin Sports Med. 2001;20(3):565–90.
27. Takahara M, Ogino T, Fukushima S, Tsuchida H, Kaneda K. Nonoperative treatment of osteochondritis dissecans of the humeral capitellum. Am J Sports Med. 1999;27(6):728–32.
28. de Graaff F, Krijnen MR, Poolman RW, Willems WJ. Arthroscopic surgery in athletes with osteochondritis dissecans of the elbow. Arthroscopy. 2011;27(7):986–93.

29. Iwasaki N, Kato H, Ishikawa J, Masuko T, Funakoshi T, Minami A. Autologous osteochondral mosaicplasty for osteochondritis dissecans of the elbow in teenage athletes: surgical technique. J Bone Joint Surg Am. 2010;92(Suppl 1 Pt):2208–16.

30. Kuwahata Y, Inoue G. Osteochondritis dissecans of the elbow managed by Herbert screw fixation. Orthopedics. 1998;21(4):449–51.

31. Takeda H, Watarai K, Matsushita T, Saito T, Terashima Y. A surgical treatment for unstable osteochondritis dissecans lesions of the humeral capitellum in adolescent baseball players. Am J Sports Med. 2002;30(5):713–7.

32. Vogt S, Siebenlist S, Hensler D, Weigelt L, Ansah P, Woertler K, et al. Osteochondral transplantation in the elbow leads to good clinical and radiologic long-term results: an 8- to 14-year follow-up examination. Am J Sports Med. 2011;39(12):2619–25.

33. van den Ende KI, McIntosh AL, Adams JE, Steinmann SP. Osteochondritis dissecans of the capitellum: a review of the literature and a distal ulnar portal. Arthroscopy. 2011;27(1):122–8.

34. Baumgarten TE, Andrews JR, Satterwhite YE. The arthroscopic classification and treatment of osteochondritis dissecans of the capitellum. Am J Sports Med. 1998;26(4):520–3.

35. Byrd JW, Jones KS. Arthroscopic surgery for isolated capitellar osteochondritis dissecans in adolescent baseball players: minimum three-year follow-up. Am J Sports Med. 2002;30(4):474–8.

36. O'Driscoll SW. The healing and regeneration of articular cartilage. J Bone Joint Surg Am. 1998;80(12):1795–812.

37. Wulf CA, Stone RM, Giveans MR, Lervick GN. Magnetic resonance imaging after arthroscopic microfracture of capitellar osteochondritis dissecans. Am J Sports Med. 2012;40(11):2549–56.

38. Schoch B, Wolf BR. Osteochondritis dissecans of the capitellum: minimum 1-year follow-up after arthroscopic debridement. Arthroscopy. 2010;26(11):1469–73.

39. Bojanic I, Ivkovic A, Boric I. Arthroscopy and microfracture technique in the treatment of osteochondritis dissecans of the humeral capitellum: report of three adolescent gymnasts. Knee Surg Sports Traumatol Arthrosc. 2006;14(5):491–6.

40. Jones KJ, Wiesel BB, Sankar WN, Ganley TJ. Arthroscopic management of osteochondritis dissecans of the capitellum: mid-term results in adolescent athletes. J Pediatr Orthop. 2010;30(1):8–13.

41. Miyake J, Masatomi T. Arthroscopic debridement of the humeral capitellum for osteochondritis dissecans: radiographic and clinical outcomes. J Hand Surg Am. 2011;36(8):1333–8.

42. Rahusen FT, Brinkman JM, Eygendaal D. Results of arthroscopic debridement for osteochondritis dissecans of the elbow. Br J Sports Med. 2006;40(12):966–9.

43. Elfeddali R, Schreuder MH, Eygendaal D. Arthroscopic elbow surgery, is it safe? J Shoulder Elbow Surg. 2013;22(5):647–52.

44. Nelson GN, Wu T, Galatz LM, Yamaguchi K, Keener JD. Elbow arthroscopy: early complications and associated risk factors. J Shoulder Elbow Surg. 2014;23(2):273–8.

45. Hennrikus WP, Miller PE, Micheli LJ, Waters PM, Bae DS. Internal fixation of unstable in situ osteochondritis dissecans lesions of the capitellum. J Pediatr Orthop. 2015;35(5):467–73.

46. Nobuta S, Ogawa K, Sato K, Nakagawa T, Hatori M, Itoi E. Clinical outcome of fragment fixation for osteochondritis dissecans of the elbow. Ups J Med Sci. 2008;113(2):201–8.

47. Kosaka M, Nakase J, Takahashi R, Toratani T, Ohashi Y, Kitaoka K, et al. Outcomes and failure factors in surgical treatment for osteochondritis dissecans of the capitellum. J Pediatr Orthop. 2013;33(7):719–24.

48. Hangody L, Fules P. Autologous osteochondral mosaicplasty for the treatment of full-thickness defects of weight-bearing joints: ten years of experimental and clinical experience. J Bone Joint Surg Am. 2003;85(Suppl):225–32.

49. Maruyama M, Takahara M, Harada M, Satake H, Takagi M. Outcomes of an open autologous osteochondral plug graft for capitellar osteochondritis dissecans: time to return to sports. Am J Sports Med. 2014;42(9):2122–7.

50. Ovesen J, Olsen BS, Johannsen HV. The clinical outcomes of mosaicplasty in the treatment of osteochondritis dissecans of the distal humeral capitellum of young athletes. J Shoulder Elbow Surg. 2011;20(5):813–8.

51. Nishimura A, Morita A, Fukuda A, Kato K, Sudo A. Functional recovery of the donor knee after autologous osteochondral transplantation for capitellar osteochondritis dissecans. Am J Sports Med. 2011;39(4):838–42.

52. Kiyoshige Y, Takagi M, Yuasa K, Hamasaki M. Closed-Wedge osteotomy for osteochondritis dissecans of the capitellum. A 7- to 12-year follow-up. Am J Sports Med. 2000;28(4):534–7.

53. Nishinaka N, Tsutsui H, Yamaguchi K, Uehara T, Nagai S, Atsumi T. Costal osteochondral autograft for reconstruction of advanced-stage osteochondritis dissecans of the capitellum. J Shoulder Elbow Surg. 2014;23(12):1888–97.

54. Shimada K, Tanaka H, Matsumoto T, Miyake J, Higuchi H, Gamo K, et al. Cylindrical costal osteochondral autograft for reconstruction of large defects of the capitellum due to osteochondritis dissecans. J Bone Joint Surg Am. 2012;94(11):992–1002.

The Stiff Painful Elbow in the Athlete

7

Abbas Rashid

Contents

Key Learning Points

- Painful elbow impingement may occur anteriorly, posteriorly or with a combination of the two. Posterior impingement can be medial, lateral or combined.
- The most common cause of impingement is osteophyte formation leading to localised synovitis.
- Posteromedial impingement may occur as a result of gradual stretching of the medial collateral ligament (Valgus extension overload).
- Elbow stiffness can be caused by a number of conditions. Consider whether the cause is extrinsic (extra-articular causes such as capsu-

lar, collateral ligament muscle contractures, HO, extra-articular malunions) or intrinsic (intra-articular adhesions, loose bodies, osteophytes, malalignment of the articular surface) or mixed (extrinsic contractures developing as a result of intrinsic pathology).

7.1   Evaluation of the Stiff Elbow

The history should include details about the patient (age, hand dominance, occupation, type of sport and level of involvement); the injury (mechanism, nature of injury, operative details including surgical approaches, type of hardware, nerve transposition, post-operative infection); the

A. Rashid (✉)
University College London Hospital, London, UK
e-mail: abbas.rashid@nhs.net

impact of current symptoms and what their functional goals are.

Patients typically complain of a combination of pain, stiffness or mechanical symptoms. It is important to determine the anatomical location of pain, where it occurs in the arc of motion (terminal vs. throughout the arc) and which phase of throwing (early acceleration vs. terminal extension). Stiffness usually refers to a loss of range of movement, can affect one or both planes of motion and may be painful or painless. It is important to determine the onset and course of the stiffness; did it come on suddenly or was there a gradual loss of range, is it progressive or relapsing, is the loss of flexion and extension the same. Mechanical symptoms such as snapping, catching or locking may accompany pain or stiffness.

The elbow is inspected for deformity, swelling and scars from previous surgery. Boney (lateral epicondyle, radiocapitellar joint, olecranon tip and medial epicondyle) and soft tissue elements (common extensor origin, lateral gutter, triceps insertion, posteromedial gutter, common flexor/pronator origin, the distal biceps tendon and lacertus fibrosus) should be palpated in a systematic manner. The elbow is taken through its active and passive range of motion, looking for disparity between the two as well as making comparison between the affected and contralateral side (throwing athletes lack terminal extension in the throwing arm) and feeling for the nature of the endpoint (hard vs. soft). Isometric muscle testing is performed by placing each of the four muscle groups (biceps, triceps, wrist extensors and wrist flexors/forearm pronators) in their maximal position of tension and testing strength against resistance. Capsulo-ligamentous stability is tested by placing the elbow in 30° of flexion and applying varus and valgus stress looking for pain and or apprehension with more specific tests for the LUCL (postero-lateral drawer test or push off test) and MCL (moving valgus stress test or milking manoeuvre). The Ulnar nerve is frequently involved with elbow pathology and should be assessed for location (if previously transposed), irritability (positive compression test or a Tinel's sign), subluxation with elbow flexion and general

sensory-motor function in the hand. Analysis of the throwing action is imperative as elbow pathology may be alleviated by minor adjustments of the throwing action or elsewhere in the kinetic chain.

Plain radiographs are obtained in orthogonal and two oblique planes, which demonstrate most boney pathology. Furthermore, elevated fat pads can help differentiate between soft tissue swelling and an effusion, which is often secondary to occult intra-articular pathology. CT permits 3D assessment of complex post-traumatic deformity and, when combined with arthrography, demonstrates soft tissue pathology such as cartilage defects, loose bodies and ligament injuries. MRI with or without arthrography can be useful in cases of suspected instability, which can present with elbow stiffness due to recurrent effusions.

If inflammatory markers are elevated in the context of previous surgery, then aspiration should be performed through the soft spot in an aseptic environment to exclude infection. Neurophysiology is useful to assess the prognosis of a recovering Ulnar nerve injury.

7.2 Post-traumatic Osteoarthritis

Traumatic damage to articular cartilage and subsequent incongruences change load distribution across the bearing surface, culminating in the development of osteoarthritis [1]. Unlike idiopathic osteoarthritis it is usually restricted to the specific area that was injured. Although rare, the pain and disability coupled with the functional demands of athletes makes it difficult to treat.

In the early stages patients present with terminal arc pain due to periarticular osteophytes and mild stiffness due to extrinsic capsular contracture. As articular degeneration then progresses, patients increasingly complain of: pain throughout the arc of motion (particularly at rest and at night) stiffness, crepitus and sometimes locking (due to loose bodies). Infection, radicular pain and CRPS also present in this manner and must be excluded [2].

The elbow is evaluated as described above. Although radiographs show larger osteophytes, loose bodies and joint space narrowing, CT arthrogram more accurately demonstrates osteophyte distribution, articular cartilage defects and capsulo-ligamentous contracture [3].

The goals of treatment are managing pain and maintaining joint mobility. The mainstay of treatment is usually non-operative and includes activity modification (minimising weight bearing or repetitive motions that place undue stress across the joint); physiotherapy; and pharmacologic treatment (oral NSAIDS or selective intra-articular corticosteroid injection).

The aim of surgery is to restore joint function and relieve pain whilst preserving the possibility of future salvage. Patients experiencing impingement are best served with open or arthroscopic osteocapsular release and joint debridement (Fig. 7.1). This involves removal of loose bodies and osteophytes, subtotal capsulectomy, selective release of the MCL to improve flexion, with transposition of the ulnar nerve if there is preoperative ulnar neuritis or flexion is limited to less than 90° (as larger flexion gains with surgery may inadvertently stretch the nerve). Patients with more advanced disease are best served with interposition arthroplasty, resection arthroplasty or partial replacement arthroplasty but these would most likely end their sporting career. Radial head resection is indicated in patients with isolated radiocapitellar osteoarthritis affecting forearm rotation, although there is a theoretical risk of increased force transmission through the ulnohumeral joint promoting early degenerative changes. Interposition arthroplasty involves removal of the radial head and interposition of autograft or allograft into the gap, thus improving lateral ligament complex tensioning and, therefore, valgus stability (although it does not improve axial stability). Partial replacement arthroplasty options include radial head replacement (which restore lateral column stability but reduce radiocapitellar contact) and radiocapitellar resurfacing (which provides valgus and axial stability, although this is a more extensive procedure). Although total joint arthroplasty provides predicable pain relief, patients are unlikely to accept the functional restrictions (limit isolated lifts to less than 10 lbs and repetitive lifts to less than 5 lbs) and the likelihood of deterioration over time necessitating revision surgery [4].

7.3　Posterolateral Impingement

This is usually due to either inflammation and hypertrophy of a synovial plica (a mesenchymal remnant from normal development) in the lateral compartment or posterolateral osteophyte formation [5, 6]. Repetitive hyperextension during the follow-through phase of throwing and swinging causes microtrauma to the plica (only occasionally present), which becomes inflamed causing

Fig. 7.1 (**a**) Arthroscopic view of Outerbridge-Kashiwagi procedure. Burring from posterior compartment into anterior compartment to excise bi-compartmental osteophytes and release capsule. (**b**) Post-op AP radiograph showing hole in olecranon fossa

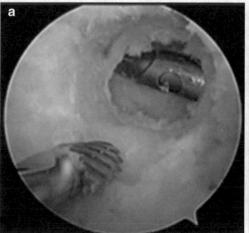
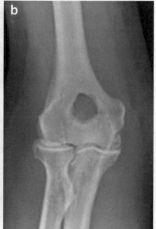

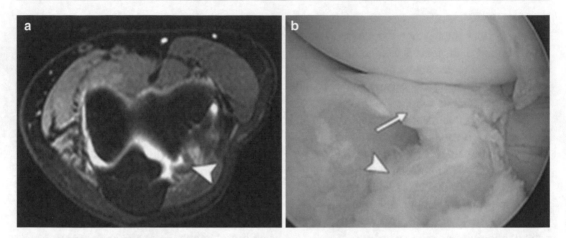

Fig. 7.2 (**a**) Axial T1 weighted fat-suppressed image showing postero-lateral plica. (**b**) Arthroscopic view of lateral compartment showing hypertrophied plica (arrow) and associated focal fibrosis (arrow head)

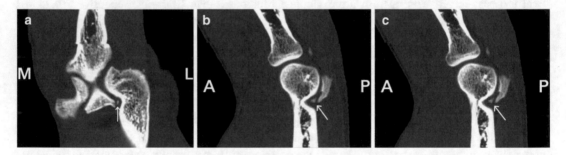

Fig. 7.3 Preoperative CT scans. The white arrows indicate an osteophyte and loose body. (**a**) Coronal view; (**b**) sagittal view; (**c**) transverse view. *M* medial, *L* lateral, *A* anterior, *P* posterior

pain (Fig. 7.2). The plica subsequently hypertrophies and gets caught on the radiocapitellar joint during movement, felt as snapping or catching, resulting in chondromalacia of the involved bony surfaces. Alternatively, repetitive hyperextension in pronation, as seen in boxers who miss punches or goalkeepers blocking a football, may result in abnormal contact between the posterolateral olecranon and the fossa resulting in osteophytes that cause pain and locking. Unlike posteromedial impingement it is not associated with any micro-instability.

Patients complain of posterolateral elbow pain in the region of the Anconeus muscle. Symptoms can be reproduced by passively flexing the pronated elbow (flexion-pronation test). Other conditions presenting with lateral-sided elbow pain (e.g. lateral epicondylitis and osteochodritis dis-

secans) need to be excluded. CT arthrogram shows articular cartilage defects and plicae, as well as osteophyte distribution (Fig. 7.3). Plicae larger than 3 mm with an irregular or nodular appearance are usually associated with symptoms [5].

Although selective corticosteroid injections offer therapeutic benefit, symptoms invariably return on return to sport. We, therefore, recommend arthroscopic excision of the plicae with debridement of chondromalacia or excision of osteophytes and or removal of loose bodies as required. Patients should refrain from throwing or swinging for approximately 6–8 weeks postoperatively, followed by a progressive throwing or swinging programme. The majority of patients can return to their previous level of sport by approximately 4–6 months. The presence of chondromalacia does not affect the functional outcome and return to sport.

7.4   Posteromedial Impingement

Repetitive overhead throwing places large valgus stresses on the elbow, 50% of which are absorbed by the MCL [7, 8]. These stresses are exacerbated by poor throwing mechanics (e.g. late trunk rotation, reduced shoulder external rotation and increased elbow flexion). This causes progressive laxity of the medial soft tissues to the extent that the normally conforming medial compartment undergoes micromotion when the elbow is forcibly extended. As a consequence, the posteromedial tip of the olecranon impinges on the medial wall of the olecranon fossa, resulting in localised synovitis manifesting as pain (Fig. 7.4) [9]. The body responds by creating osteophytes on the posteromedial tip of the olecranon in order to restore stability. These can fracture and lodge in the posteromedial gutter causing mechanical symptoms such as locking, clicking or snapping.

Patients complain of posteromedial elbow pain during ball release when the elbow nears terminal extension. If, however, the patient experiences medial pain in the early acceleration phase of throwing there may be concurrent MCL insufficiency. On examination there is usually focal tenderness over the posteromedial gutter, with loss of terminal extension and MCL laxity (although this does not have to be present for the condition to develop). Symptoms can be reproduced by placing the elbow in 20–30° of flexion while forcing the elbow into terminal extension and applying a valgus stress (Valgus Extension Overload Test). Other causes of medial elbow pain (e.g. flexor-pronator tendinopathy, medial epicondylitis, ulnar neuritis) must be excluded. MRI is useful early on in the disease process as it may show insertional tendinopathy at the medial border of the triceps with subenthesial bone marrow oedema in the olecranon [10]. However, in advanced cases CT arthrogram shows obvious bony and articular changes to the posterior trochlea and olecranon along with posteromedial gut-

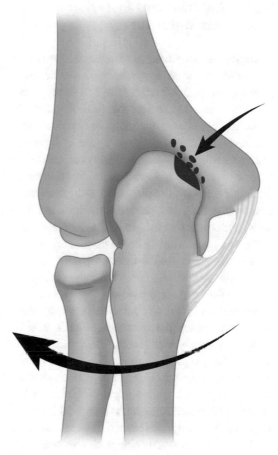

Fig. 7.4 Valgus extension overload resulting in posteromedial impingement

ter synovitis. Compression forces through the lateral compartment often result in corresponding imaging abnormalities in the lateral compartment.

Non-operative treatment consists of NSAIDS, selective corticosteroid injections and active rest (including rest from throwing), cuff strengthening, flexor-pronator strengthening, and an interval throwing mechanics programme. If, however, these measures fail we recommend arthroscopic excision of the olecranon spur (which should be restricted to less than 8 mm to avoid potentiating any MCL insufficiency), microfracture of areas of cartilage loss (typically in the posteromedial trochlea) and loose body excision, with or without MCL reefing or autograft reconstruction.

7.5   Anterior and Posterior Impingement

Posterior impingement in athletes is usually due to olecranon stress fracture, with two separate patterns seen. Tip fractures are due to repetitive loads induced by the forceful pull of triceps or from impaction of a hypertrophic olecranon into the olecranon fossa, commonly seen in throwers. Fractures of the middle third, however, are due to a repetitive valgus force across the olecranon from impaction of the olecranon within the fossa, commonly seen in weightlifters throwing athletes, gymnasts and weight lifters. Patients complain of posterior elbow pain during the acceleration and follow-through phases, throwing with limitation of terminal extension. Examination reveals tenderness directly over the olecranon and pain on resisted elbow extension. Almost all cases have concurrent MCL and or medial epicondyle avulsion. Plain radiographs confirm the diagnosis, although in some instances findings may be subtle, such as periosteal reaction. If there is a high clinical suspicion in the context of normal radiographs then MRI is necessary (and can help exclude a triceps tendon tear/avulsion). Treatment begins with 6–8 weeks of

rest from the inciting activity, followed by a graduated programme of sport-specific rehabilitation. Failing this we advise debridement of the non-union and internal fixation with bone grafting.

Anterior impingement is usually due to coronoid osteophytes and is most commonly seen in boxers. It can occur as a result of coronoid fracture malunion secondary to elbow hyperextension or shearing forces imparted through the trochlea with a posteriorly directed force through the forearm such as in close quarters fighting or pushing off from a clinch [11, 12]. Although traditionally associated with recurrent elbow instability, they do occasionally lead to hypertrophic malunion and fibrous non-union in a prominent position, thus blocking elbow flexion. Plain radiographs and CT arthrogram are diagnostic (Fig. 7.5). Treatment consists of excising the non-union and allograft fixation to recreate the coronoid in order to avoid instability.

7.6   Post-traumatic Stiffness

A stiff elbow is one that cannot achieve flexion of 30–130° or pronation of 50° and supination of 50° (although loss of supination is less well toler-

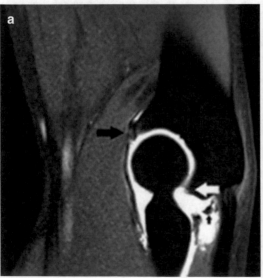
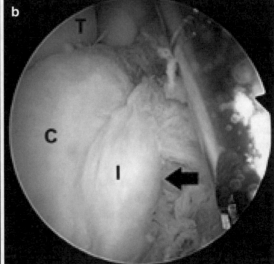

Fig. 7.5 (a) T2 weighted MRI scan demonstrating coronoid osteophyte in the anterior compartment (thick black arrow), an impingement lesion at the tip of the olecranon (white arrow) and a loose body (small black arrow). (b) Arthroscopic view of coronoid osteophyte and impingement lesion. *T* trochlea, *C* coronoid, *I* impingement lesion

ated, as shoulder abduction cannot compensate for it) [13, 14]. Stiffness in athletes is usually due to trauma (fractures, dislocations, soft tissue and head injury and surgery) due to one or a combination of arthrosis, soft tissue contracture, heterotopic ossification and non-union or malunion [13]. It is classified by Kay on the combination of elements impeding elbow motion (type I = soft tissue contracture, type II = soft tissue contracture with ossification, type III = undisplaced articular fracture with soft tissue contracture, type IV = displaced articular fracture with soft tissue contracture and type V = bony bars); and by Morrey on the anatomic location of the pathology (extra-articular causes such as capsular, collateral ligament muscle contractures, HO, extra-articular malunions), intrinsic (intra-articular adhesions, loose bodies, osteophytes, malignment of the articular surface) or mixed (extrinsic contractures developing as a result of intrinsic pathology). It is important to consider the hidden cause of instability such as neural causes (usually from entrapment of the ulnar nerve) and instability.

Soft tissue contracture Any insult to the elbow that results in bleeding, oedema and granulation tissue formation. The net effect is upregulation of TGF-β in ligaments and soft tissues, stimulating an increase in myofibroblasts and α-smooth muscle actin resulting in capsular fibrosis and subsequent joint contracture. The risk can be minimised by splinting the elbow in full extension (which creates sufficient pressure within the tissues to minimise bleeding and resist extravasation of fluid) and using CPM immediately postoperatively (which drives fluids away from the joint and peri-articular tissues, thus halting the cascade of events leading to soft tissue contractures). Post-traumatic stiffness is typically not painful and endpoints are soft [15].

HO This is the inappropriate formation of lamellar bone in the soft tissues. This requires osteogenic precursor cells, an inductive agent and a conducive environment. It is histologically identical to native bone but is more metabolically active and doesn't have a true periosteal layer.

HO restricts movement by causing generalised stiffness and less often radio-ulnar synostosis limiting rotation (Fig. 7.6). 3% of simple elbow dislocations and 30% of fracture dislocations are complicated by HO. Approximately 5–10% of patients with closed head injury and spinal cord injury form HO as they have higher circulating levels of osteblastic growth factors. Those patients with head injury and concurrent elbow trauma have a rate of 76–89% development of HO. Additional risk factors include two-incision distal biceps repair, elbow arthroscopy and multiple surgery within 7–14 days after trauma [13]. HO is classified by Hastings & Graham: class I = HO not causing functional limitation and, therefore, clinically insignificant; class II = HO with functional limitation with IIA representing ulnohumeral limitation with less than a 100° flexion arc, IIB representing forearm rotation limitation

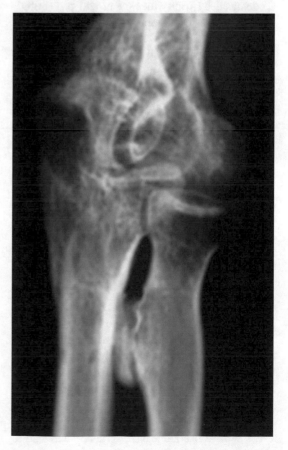

Fig. 7.6 Oblique radiograph showing post-traumatic radio-ulnar synostosis

with less than a 100° rotation arc and IIC representing limitation in both planes; class III = ankylosis that prevents flexion, rotation or both.

Prevention of HO is based on disrupting signalling pathways (NSAIDS inhibit COX, thus reducing prostaglandin levels, which are partly responsible for inducing HO), altering the progenitor cells (adjuvant radiotherapy stops stem cells differentiating into osteoblasts) or modifying the osteogenic environment (post-operative etidronate interferes with calcification of osteoid in HO by inhibiting angiogenesis). HO presents within 12 weeks of an inciting event as localised soft tissue swelling, warmth and tenderness (often mistaken for infection, cellulitis or thrombophlebitis) and endpoints are hard. Surgery can only be undertaken in symptomatic cases when radiographic maturity is achieved (measured by time since onset and physiological activity). On plain radiographs a cloudy peri-articular density is usually seen several weeks after injury and maturity is indicated by smooth well demarcated cortical margins and defined trabecular markings, generally about 3–6 months after its onset.

Extra-articular malunion The lateral column of the distal humerus is curved anteriorly with the lateral epicondyle translated anteriorly with respect to the humeral diaphysis. Failure to restore this relationship (e.g. by using a straight plate rather than an anatomically pre-contoured plate on the lateral column or bridging a highly comminuted fracture that subsequently shortens and obscures the coronoid or olecranon fossae) may reduce the available space for the coronoid and olecranon to engage their respective fossae. In treating this entity, the fossae should be cleared of HO, scar and implants then a burr used to deepen the hole or even fenestrate it permitting an osteocapsular release. If this does not work then extra-articular osteotomy is an option.

Intra-articular malunion Uneven articular surfaces with subsequent incongruency can lead to stiffness by arthrosis. Malunited radial head fractures limit rotation but can be treated successfully by radial head excision (except in Essex-Loprsti injuries and terrible triad injuries). Malunited intra-articular fractures of the proximal ulna limit flexion-extension and are treated with restoration of the trochlear notch. Coronoid malunited anterior shear fractures of the capitellum or trochlea can be treated with osteotomy and capsular release.

Non-union Non-union tends to occur at the supracondylar level leading to motion at the non-union site and ankylosis of the joint. These can be addressed with excision of the non-union, fixation with bone grafting, capsulectomy and an intense rehabilitation programme. Non-union of proximal ulna fractures (olecranon fractures, olecranon osteotomy, iatrogenic fractures during TEA and Monteggia fractures) are less common, most of which are successfully managed non-operatively especially iatrogenic fractures during TEA.

Surgical treatment involves excision of non-union, revision fixation with bone grafting with the addition that the coronoid should be included in the fixation if large or reconstructed if small. Olecranon non-union can also result from simple olecranon fractures or osteotomy. Radial head non-unions are extremely uncommon. Those treated operatively, however, often lead to stiffness through broken or loose implants causing limited rotation or a block to flexion. Removal of implants and excision of the radial head will usually solve this problem.

7.7   Treatment of Elbow Stiffness

Non-operative treatments Non-operative treatment is useful in contractures of 6 months' duration or less. Options include active mobilisation with physiotherapy guidance, static and dynamic splinting, serial casting and manipulation.

Physiotherapy is the mainstay of treatment in the early phases. This should include efforts to control pain and swelling. Active mobilisation exercises are recommended in preference to passive stretch. See the chapter on elbow rehabilitation for more details.

Some practitioners recommend the use of static splints to apply stress relaxation force to the tissues, which is sequentially increased as motion is achieved and can produce a 25–43° increase in the arc of motion. Although more cumbersome than dynamic splints, they offer more comfort due to the inherent stress relaxation of the tissues. Dynamic splints apply a constant prolonged force to the tissues as additional motion is achieved and have been shown to increase the arc of motion by 39%. Once a stiff elbow is pain free, the splint can be applied at night with serial increases in the tension of its adjustable spring. However, co-contraction of the elbow flexors and extensors due to constant tension on the soft tissues often causes more pain and discomfort resulting in non-compliance. Zander and Healy have shown that elbow flexion contracture can be reduced by 33° with the use of serial casting. Manipulation can be beneficial within the first 6 weeks but risks include reports of transient ulnar neuropathies, peri-articular fracture and HO [13].

Surgical treatment Young age, stiffness secondary to arthrosis and intervention more than 1 year from the onset of symptoms (more contracted the muscles and tendons) are related to poor surgical outcomes. Arthroscopy can be used to address both bony blocks to motion and soft tissue contracture, although decreased intra-articular volume makes access more difficult and iatrogenic neurovascular injury more likely. Good results have been reported with open and arthroscopic releases with previous ulnar nerve transposition being a contraindication to arthroscopy [13].

The approach depends upon the plane of elbow contracture, the location and extent of HO, location of previous incisions and need for ulnar nerve decompression. The lateral approach (column procedure) is preferred for radio-capitellar articular pathology but also permits anterior and posterior capsule contracture release. It is usually done with a concurrent medial approach to decompress the ulnar nerve if required (if there is concurrent scarring from the MCL contracture that forms the bed of the cubital tunnel or if the patient has pre-operative flex-

ion limited to less than 90°, as gains in flexion may stretch the nerve). The medial over the top approach is preferred for ulno-humeral articular pathology and allows release of the MCL and ulnar nerve. The main risk of this procedure is that the radial nerve is at risk at the depth of the exposure on the far side anteriorly. Furthermore, it may not be effective when there is extensive articular involvement. The anterior approach is useful when HO is located anteromedial to the radial head or along the ulno-humeral articulation within Brachialis. This approach permits visualisation of the entire anterior capsule and median nerve for safe excision of HO. HO resulting in proximal radio ulnar synostosis is best treated with radial head resection just distal to the synostosis and can increase arc of rotation from 0 to 98° (Fig. 7.6). Regardless of the approach used, every attempt is made to preserve the lateral collateral ligament and the anterior oblique band if the MCL, as it enhances rehabilitation and avoids instability. The most common complications are neuropathies, infection, recurrence and HO. Injection of botulinum toxin A into the elbow flexors at the time of contracture release or even up to 2 months postoperatively when patients fail to progress, can improve range of motion [13].

Q&A
Q1: How would you assess the patient presenting with a stiff and painful elbow?

The assessment starts by taking a careful history from the patient detailing when and where the experience the pain, what makes it worse and what makes it better. If the elbow is stiff is this progressive or intermittent? Record careful the detail of any trauma. A careful examination should be conducted working through the differential diagnosis. Imaging with Xrays, CT or MRI may be helpful to confirm the diagnosis and for treatment planning.

Q2: What are the causes of elbow stiffness?

Stiffness in athletes is usually due to trauma resulting in one or a combination of arthrosis, soft tissue contracture, heterotopic ossification and non-union or malunion. It is classified according to the structure that is impeding elbow motion and the type of pathology. It is important to consider the hidden cause of instability such as neural causes (usually from entrapment of the ulnar nerve) and instability.

Q3: What is the best treatment for an elbow that is stiff within 6 months of an injury.

The first objective is to determine the cause of the stiffness. If there is no evidence of a mechanical block to movement then the first line treatment should be physiotherapy with the aim of controlling pain and swelling and encouraging active mobilisation exercises. Careful serial documentation of the range of movement measured with a goniometer will show evidence of progress which can encourage the patient.

References

1. Wysocki RW, Cohen MS. Primary osteoarthritis and posttraumatic arthritis of the elbow. Hand Clin. 2011;27(2):131–7.
2. Cheung EV, Adams R, Morrey BF. Primary osteoarthritis of the elbow: current treatment options. J Am Acad Orthop Surg. 2008;16(2):77–87.
3. Rettig LA, Hastings H II, Feinberg JR. Primary osteoarthritis of the elbow: lack of radiographic evidence for morphologic predisposition, results of operative debridement at intermediate follow-up, and basis for a new radiographic classification system. J Shoulder Elbow Surg. 2008;17(1):97–105.
4. Sears BW, Puskas GJ, Morrey ME, Sanchez-Sotelo J, Morrey BF. Posttraumatic elbow arthritis in the young adult: evaluation and management. J Am Acad Orthop Surg. 2012;20(11):704–14.
5. Kim DH, Gambardella RA, Elattrache NS, Yocum LA, Jobe FW. Arthroscopic treatment of posterolateral elbow impingement from lateral synovial plicae in throwing athletes and golfers. Am J Sports Med. 2006;34(3):438–44.
6. Valkering KP, van der Hoeven H, Pijnenburg BC. Posterolateral elbow impingement in professional boxers. Am J Sports Med. 2008;36(2):328–32.
7. Wilson FD, Andrews JR, Blackburn TA, McCluskey G. Valgus extension overload in the pitching elbow. Am J Sports Med. 1983;11(2):83–8.
8. Hotchkiss RN, Weiland AJ. Valgus stability of the elbow. J Orthop Res. 1987;5:372–7.
9. Limpisvasti O, ElAttrache NS, Jobe FW. Understanding shoulder and elbow injuries in baseball. J Am Acad Orthop Surg. 2007;15(3):139–47.
10. Cohen SB, Valko C, Zoga A, Dodson CC, Ciccotti MG. Posteromedial elbow impingement: magnetic resonance imaging findings in overhead throwing athletes and results of arthroscopic treatment. Arthroscopy. 2011;27(10):1364–70.
11. Robinson PM, Loosemore M, Watts AC. Boxer's elbow: internal impingement of the coronoid and olecranon process. A report of seven cases. J Shoulder Elbow Surg. 2017;26(3):376–81. https://doi.org/10.1016/j.jse.2016.09.035. Epub 2016 Nov 18.
12. Liu SH, Henry M, Bowen R. Complications of type I coronoid fractures in competitive athletes: report of two cases and review of the literature. J Shoulder Elbow Surg. 1996;5(3):223–7.
13. Evans PJ, Nandi S, Maschke S, Hoyen HA, Lawton JN. Prevention and treatment of elbow stiffness. J Hand Surg Am. 2009;34(4):769–78.
14. Morrey BF, Askew LJ, Chao EY. A biomechanical study of normal functional elbow motion. J Bone Joint Surg Am. 1981;63(6):872–7.
15. Lindenhovius AL, Jupiter JB. The posttraumatic stiff elbow: a review of the literature. J Hand Surg Am. 2007;32(10):1605–23.

Tendon Injuries Around the Elbow

8

Jeremy Granville-Chapman and Adam C. Watts

Contents

J. Granville-Chapman (✉)
Consultant Upper Limb Surgeon at Frimley Health
NHS Foundation Trust, Heatherwood and Wexham
Park Hospital, Slough, UK
e-mail: jgchapman@doctors.org.uk

A. C. Watts
Wrightington Hospital Upper Limb Unit,
Wrightington, UK
e-mail: adam.watts@elbowdoc.co.uk

Key Learning Points

1. Be aware of the incidence of elbow tendinopathy and its impact on time off work and sport.
2. Understand the current basic science understanding of tendinopathy.
3. Recognise that corticosteroid injections are not indicated, and are harmful, in elbow tendinopathy.
4. Be able to differentiate clinically between acute reactive tendinopathy and chronic degenerative tendinopathy and recognise how this affects management and prognosis.
5. Be able to prescribe an evidence-based management plan for elbow tendon pathologies, including advising on the natural history, the role of therapy, injections, electrotherapy's and surgery.
6. For tendon rupture, understand the relative roles of conservative and surgical management.

8.1 The Normal Tendon

Normal tendon is a composite viscoelastic biomaterial that transmits muscle contraction force to bone. The principal matrix protein is Type 1 collagen—a helical structure composed of long, staggered, cross-linked proteins, that functions much like a rope in resisting tensile forces. A hierarchical structure organises these collagen bundles into crimped fibrils that are aligned to stress. These crimped fibrils absorb early stress exerted on the tendon and produce the 'toe region' of the tendon load-deformation curve. Other collagen subtypes may also be present, as well as proteoglycan and glycoprotein molecules. The cellular component is formed of tenocytes: these fibroblast-like cells are responsible for the maintenance of the matrix.

The insertion of tendon into bone is termed the 'enthesis'. This region comprises a transition from tendon substance to bone, via fibrocartilage and mineralised fibrocartilage. The fibrocartilage regions assist load distribution across the changing tissues. A tendon's blood supply may be rich if it's covered by a paratenon (e.g. Achilles tendon), or it may rely on diffusion from synovial fluid and segmental supply from vinculae (e.g. flexor tendons in the hand). There may be 'watershed areas' of blood supply where tissue is vulnerable to ischaemia.

As for all biomaterials, a constant (albeit slow) turnover recycles the matrix and repairs damage. Matrix breakdown is effected by 'matrix metalloproteinase' enzymes (MMPs) (which cleave collagen) and 'a disintegrin and metalloproteinase with thrombospondin motifs' (ADAMTS) (which degrade proteoglycans). 'Tissue inhibitors of metalloproteinase' (TIMPs) balance the rate of degradation. The co-ordination of this turnover in tendons remains incompletely understood, but the concept of the 'neuro-mast cell unit' has been proposed that is thought to play a role in the development of tendinopathy [1]. Such a balance between degradation and repair is key to normal tendon homeostasis. Increased loading will prompt an adaptive anabolic response in the biomaterial and this is desirable. Overuse or abnormal loading can, however, cause tissue damage and a neurogenic response.

Collagen fibres stiffen with age and crimping reduces. This explains the epidemiology of tendinopathy, with peak incidence in patients aged 35–55 years. Figure 8.1 below is a Stress strain curve for a tendon. It illustrates the 'toe zone' where the tendons initially uncramp during loading before entering the linear zone between 2 and 4% strain. Beyond this level, micro or partial tendon injury will occur. Physiological loading occurs in the

Fig. 8.1 Stress Strain curve for a healthy tendon (black solid curve) and an ageing stiff tendon (red dashed line). Modified from: An Introduction to Biomechanics and Mechanobiology. M Doblaré, J Merodio. Universities of Zaragoza and Polytechnic University of Madrid. 2015

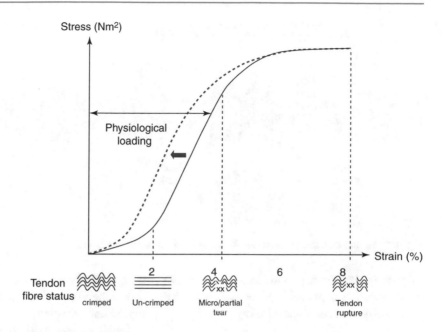

0–4% strain region. With ageing (red dashed line), the fibres stiffen and crimp less effectively. This reduces the toe zone and moves the curve to the left. This renders the ageing tendon vulnerable to micro and partial tears during physiological loading.

8.2   The Pathology of Tendinopathy in General

Most cases of tendinopathy occur at, or near to, the fibrocartilage region of the enthesis—an area that experiences higher stress, is less well vascularised and is exposed to shear and compressive forces. Biopsy of painful tendons demonstrates disorganised matrix, vessel proliferation and altered cellularity (increased and decreased). Inflammatory cells are rarely present, leading to the term 'tendinopathy', rather than 'tendinitis' [2]. There are increased levels of type III collagen, fibronectin and tenascin C levels (molecules associated with healing). Fibrocartilage proteoglycans are also found, suggesting an adaptation to abnormal loading (shear or compression). A catch-all term used to characterise tendinopathy: 'angio-fibroblastic hyperplasia' was coined by Nirschl [2].

Despite the prevalence of tendinopathy, only recently was a convincing proposal for the continuum from normal tendon to chronic degeneration proposed. Cook and Purdham

integrated histolopathology, clinical and animal data to suggest this model (Fig. 8.2). Three overlapping stages were proposed, producing two clinically distinct entities for treatment and prognosis [3].

8.2.1   Reactive Tendinopathy

The first stage is reactive tendinopathy; this involves a proliferative response of the matrix to overload (burst of training) or direct trauma. The proteoglycan component of the matrix increases and these hydrophilic compounds lead to the matrix swelling with water. The collagen structure remains largely intact. Proteoglycan accumulation can begin only a few hours after overloading or trauma to the tendon: this may represent a protective attempt by the tendon to resist sudden increases in load demand. The reactive tendon can return to normal state if the trigger is removed. MRI will show increased tendon diameter and a slight increase in signal on T2 imaging (increased water). Ultrasound will show intact collagen fibrils with hypoechogenic substance between fibrils.

In clinical terms, this stage is seen in a younger patient who has either sustained a direct blow to a tendon, or an increased intensity of athletic training. However, it is also considered possible that underuse

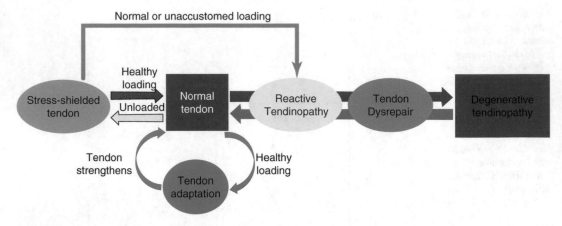

Fig. 8.2 Tendon Pathology continuum. Redrawn from Cook and Purdam [3]

of a tendon may predispose to reactive tendinopathy after return to only normal levels of loading, through structural decline and stress shielding.

8.2.2 Tendon Disrepair

The second stage occurs as the reactive tendon attempts repair. There is considerably increased matrix production, resulting in both collagen and proteoglycan synthesis. Tendon architecture becomes disrupted by proteoglycans. Changes seem to be more focal and varied. Vascular and neuronal ingrowth occurs. T2 MRI demonstrates increased signal and tendon swelling. Ultrasound reveals collagen disruption, focal areas of hypo-echogenicity and neovascularisation.

In clinical terms, this stage will have lasted longer than reactive tendinopathy and will have more focal signs on examination and imaging. It remains possible for resolution to normal tendon to occur if the loading environment is optimised.

8.2.3 Degenerative Tendinopathy

The end stage of the continuum is degenerative tendinopathy. It is here that the angiofibroblastic hyperplasia will be seen. In chronic cases, there is evidence of apoptosis as 'tenocyte exhaustion' results in abortion of attempted healing. This leads to hypocellular collagen voids within the substance of the tendon, full of vessels and matrix debris. It is probably these areas that render the

degenerate tendon at risk of rupture. Ultrasound shows the varied stages of tendinopathy, the disrupted and depleted collagen and an abundance of blood vessels. MRI shows increased size and focal areas of increased T2 signal change in the tendon substance.

The typical middle-aged sportsman, who will describe a chronic, but waxing and waning symptom profile related to training intensity illustrates this stage. The patient is likely to have focal areas of tenderness and/or nodules in the tendon. Once this stage is reached, there is little capacity for spontaneous resolution and the tendon remains at risk for rupture. A study by Tallon and colleagues demonstrated significantly greater degeneration in ruptured tendons, compared to tendinopathic tendons; and both were significantly more degenerate than asymptomatic control tendons [4].

8.3 The Relationship Between Pathology and Pain in Tendinopathy

Many patients, who have never experienced symptoms of tendinopathy, sustain tendon rupture with degenerative tendons found at surgery. Why some develop pain is unclear [5], but the notion that inflammation produces the pain has largely lost support since Nirschl's work. Many treatment strategies focus on improving the tendon biology and architecture and, through this, hope to improve the pain patients experience.

Tenocytes in tendinopathy have been shown to produce increased levels of Substance P, a neurotransmitter in the glutamate pathway [6]. A recent animal model of overuse tendinopathy further demonstrated that Substance P, a vasodilator, accelerated the vascular processes seen in tendinopathy.

8.3.1 Treatment Strategies in Tendinopathy

As our understanding of pathology improves, so treatments evolve. Numerous treatments have been examined, but disappointingly few are supported by robust evidence. Steroid injections, formerly a mainstay of conservative therapy, have now been shown to prolong the natural history of tennis elbow [7], to have a dose dependent toxic effect on tenocytes and to confound the early beneficial effect of physiotherapy. Despite this they continue to be given in practice.

It is important to assess in which stage of the continuum of tendinopathy a patient lies: if in the reactive tendinopathy or early tendon disrepair stages, there is good scope for spontaneous resolution if the precipitating activity is ceased. As such, something simple like altering training plans or increasing rest periods may be all that is required. The majority of patients who present to the specialist, however, are in chronic stages of tendinopathy. Recalcitrant sufferers are unlikely to improve with just cessation of the original trigger and require a more specific programme.

8.4 Common Extensor Origin

Tennis elbow is common with a prevalence of up to 3% [8]. Up to 15% of repetitive task workers experience tennis elbow [9]. It is most common in the fourth to the sixth decades of life [10]. While tennis elbow occurs in up to 40% of tennis players, the majority of patients do not of course play tennis [11]. Ten to 30% of sufferers take an absence from work (mean 12 weeks off) with obvious financial implications [12]. The dominant arm is affected in 74% of cases. Several studies support the notion that, for the majority

of patients, symptomatic tendinopathy is a self-limiting condition [13, 14]. Approximately 85% of patients can expect symptom resolution within a year from presentation.

Most patients present with a history of gradually increasing activity-related pain. In some, pain later becomes constant. Any history of repetitive activities in the limb is relevant. Pain is felt over the lateral elbow and may radiate along the extensor compartment of the forearm. Provoking manoeuvres usually include resisted wrist and middle finger extension with the elbow extended (the extensor carpi radialis brevis tendon inserts into the base of the middle finger metacarpal), and gripping forcefully or twisting objects. The lateral epicondyle, especially over the ECRB and EDC origins will normally be tender and may be swollen. Grip strength will be reduced secondary to pain.

Other pathologies should of course be considered. Elbow pathology may mimic tendinopathy (plica, synovitis, osteochondritis dissecans, arthritis and postero-lateral rotatory instability). Entrapment neuropathy of the posterior interosseous nerve can cause pain just distal to the lateral epicondyle. Typically, this radiates down the forearm and is made worse by repeated resisted supination. Radicular pain due to cervical nerve entrapment should also be excluded.

In many cases, imaging is not required. Plain radiography will show bony spurs in up to 20% of cases; they will also highlight osteoarthritis and previous trauma. Magnetic resonance and ultrasound scans are useful in the presence of diagnostic doubt [15], with the usual cautions surrounding observer experience for ultrasound assessment [16].

8.4.1 Tennis Elbow Treatment

The majority of patients improve over 12 months, although some experience symptoms for longer [17]. Initial focus should be on achieving rapid and enduring symptom relief using the least invasive effective method. For those who fail to improve, increasingly invasive treatments become appropriate. A host of different treatments have been tried, often in combination, to improve the symptoms of elbow tendinopathy. This section covers the more common interventions.

8.4.1.1 Physiotherapy

Eccentric training is in vogue for tendinopathy management. It is thought to stimulate collagen production by tenocytes, to moderate proteoglycan proliferation and to improve collagen cross-linking and alignment [18]. Since Alfredson proposed it in 1998, clinical efficacy has been demonstrated in several Achilles tendinopathy studies [19] and ultrasound follow-up has provided evidence of improved tendon structure in the long-term [20]. Data also exist to support eccentric exercises in tennis elbow patients. Individual protocols vary, but most involve twice-daily eccentric strengthening exercises, with or without additional stretching or massage therapy. Programmes generally last 12 weeks. A study comparing daily stretching with eccentric training demonstrated improved grip strength and complete relief of pain in 86% in those undertaking the eccentric programme [21]. Another eccentric programme by Crosier and colleagues demonstrated significantly improved grip and abolition of pain, coupled with normal ultrasound find-ings in 48% of the eccentric training group versus only 28% in those undertaking a standard regime [22].

Physiotherapy has been shown to outperform corticosteroid injection at time points greater than 6 weeks and is significantly superior at 12 months, where steroid injection fares worse than no treatment [14] (Fig. 8.3 below).

A recent systematic review supported these individual study findings [23].

Progressive stretching is also commonly employed in tennis elbow [10]. Pienimaki undertook a small comparative study between exercise with stretching and ultrasound [24]. The course lasted 6–8 weeks and physiotherapy improved pain but not grip over ultrasound. At 3 years, the same physiotherapy cohort enjoyed less pain, fewer further treatments and fewer days off work.

Movement with mobilisation has shown short-term effect in reducing pain and improving grip at 13 weeks, but longer duration has not been shown. Another recent review of various therapy combinations in tennis elbow reported short-term benefit of add-on cervical and thoracic spine manipulation, suggesting that improved analgesia facilitated more vigorous exercise rehabilitation [25].

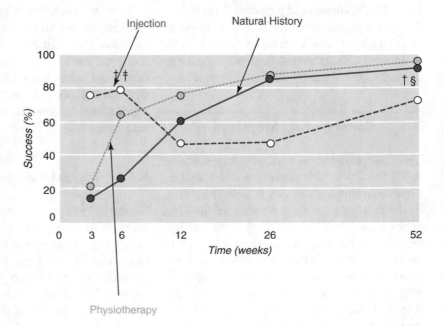

Fig. 8.3 Comparison between steroid injection, physiotherapy alone and "wait and watch" treatment from a randomized controlled trial. Red line: those receiving no treatment. Blue dashed line: those receiving corticosteroid injection. Turquoise dashed line: those receiving Physiotherapy [14]

8.4.1.2 Bracing and Orthotics

Bracing has been used to 'offload' the tendon origin. In one RCT comparing bracing with steroid injection, Jensen showed that bracing was as effective as steroid at 6 weeks [26]. Another study compared placebo bracing, unbraced controls and an off-the-shelf orthotic and showed no difference in outcomes between groups [27]. A Cochrane review in 2002 suggested that further study was required to clarify the role of bracing in tennis elbow. More recently, a wrist brace outperformed a forearm strap in a randomised trial [28]. Overall, the evidence is weak for bracing in tennis elbow, but it is possible that some treatment effect exists and it is unlikely to be harmful.

8.4.1.3 Electrotherapies

A systematic review in 2014 assessed 20 randomised controlled trials and 2 systematic reviews covering electrophysical therapies in the treatment of tennis elbow [29]. Ultrasound was supported by moderate evidence for effect over placebo at mid-term follow up. In the short-term, laser therapy was supported by moderate evidence over plyometric exercise, but was inferior to ultrasound and friction massage. Longer-term effect (beyond 3 months) has not been shown, and pooled data in Bisset's systematic review of 2005 showed no treatment effect from either modality [30].

Extracorporeal shock wave therapy (ESW) has been assessed in two good-quality, placebo-controlled, blinded trials. No improvement was found with ESW, but side effects (mostly redness or bruising) were worse in the ESW-treated cohorts [31, 32]. A Cochrane review of ESW in tennis elbow reported "Platinum level evidence that ESW provides little or no benefit in lateral elbow pain" [33].

8.4.1.4 Injection Therapies

For many years a mainstay of conservative treatment, recent work has highlighted the harmful medium and longer term effect of corticosteroid in tennis elbow. Smidt et al. compared ultrasound, friction and exercise, with corticosteroid injection or no treatment control [14]. At 6 weeks, the steroid group had improved the most, with therapy improving slightly more than controls. By 3 months however, therapy and steroid groups were equal. By 12 months, a reversal had occurred, and therapy and no treatment were significantly better than steroid injection. This finding has been supported by a systematic review into corticosteroid injections in tennis elbow [34]. Further, a recent study has refuted the notion that a steroid injection enables physiotherapy: showing that a corticosteroid injection negated the short-term beneficial effect of physiotherapy [35]. Another recent study contributed further evidence of the harmful effect of steroid injections, by demonstrating a dose-related tenocyte death rate in response to steroid injection. Steroid injection is not, therefore, indicated to facilitate active rehabilitation, it prolongs the natural history of tennis elbow and should be avoided.

8.5 Botulinum Toxin Injection

A placebo-controlled trial has shown no benefit of Botulinum Toxin A (Botox) in chronic tennis elbow patients at 3 months [36]. Another study, comparing Botox to corticosteroid injection, showed that Botox produced more weakness, but inferior pain relief at 4 weeks [37]. A systematic review has pooled data from four randomised trials with at least one pain outcome measure. Overall a beneficial effect on pain was reported, but there was no improvement in grip strength [38]. Botulinum toxin has not been compared with autologous blood injections.

8.5.1 Hyaluronic Acid

In a large, placebo-controlled trail in athletes with LE of more than 3 months' duration, two doses of Hyaluronic acid (HA) outperformed placebo in all measures out to the 1-year endpoint [39]. HA afforded a return to sport at a mean of 18 days versus no return in the placebo group.

8.5.2 Acupuncture

How acupuncture achieves a clinical improvement in pain remains controversial. A Cochrane review in 2013 found four randomised trials assessing acupuncture in tennis elbow. Overall, it is possible that acupuncture yields some improvement over placebo in the immediate and short-term (2–8 weeks), but no benefit beyond 3 months has been shown.

8.5.3 Autologous Blood Products and Platelet Rich Plasma

Platelet-rich-plasma (PRP) describes a concentrated fraction of the patient's blood. Most techniques involve: peripheral blood harvest (30 ml from a venous cannula), centrifuge separation of red cells and plasma from the platelet-rich component (within the buffy coat), local anaesthetic field block of the affected region and injection of the PRP (approx. 3 ml) by a peppering needle technique into the affected tendon origin. It is possible that, by introduction of this concentrated mixture of platelets and their growth factors to the site of tendinopathy, healing will be improved and symptoms resolve. Variability between company preparation systems makes it difficult to compare different PRP preparations and the evidence is dominated by case series, but prospective controlled trials have been undertaken and a recent Cochrane review assessed these studies [40]. This reported a possible marginal short-term pain benefit of questionable clinical impact, but overall there was inadequate evidence to support the use of PRP. Since this analysis, however, a larger RCT (230 patients) has compared PRP with needling; both groups receiving a standard physiotherapy regime [41]. While both groups improved equally at 3 months, PRP was significantly superior in treatment success rate (83.9% vs. 68.3%) and pain reduction (70.9% without significant pain vs. 46.0%) at 6 months. Unfortunately, the follow-up rate at only 51% at 6 months degrades the impact of this study.

Autologous blood injection (ABI) involves simply the injection of a small volume of blood. An RCT compared ABI (3 ml) to PRP (3 ml) injection; with both groups receiving the same physiotherapy regime [42]. PRP was marginally superior to ABI in reducing pain and this was significant at 6 weeks. Functional scores improved to a similar degree in both groups. Another RCT compared PRP and ABI in chronic cases and reported 6-month outcome scores [43]. Success rates were similar (66% PRP and 72% ABI) and overall 70% avoided surgery.

8.5.4 Autologous Tenocyte Injection

Autologous tenocyte injection aims to bring healthy housekeeping cells to the degenerate, hypocellular tendon. The process involves percutaneous biopsy under local anaesthetic of healthy tenocytes from a patella tendon. These cells are cultured in laboratory conditions and the tenocytes separated by flow cytometry. Under US guidance, the tenocytes are injected into the common extensor origin. Wang and colleagues have reported on a pilot study of 20 patients with recalcitrant chronic severe tennis elbow [44]. Patients demonstrated marked improvement in pain, qDASH, grip strength and MRI features at 12 months. Only one patient underwent surgery. A follow-up study suggested enduring benefit in these cases [45]. Further comparative studies will clarify the role of this expensive, but potentially promising technique.

8.5.5 Traumatic Avulsion

This is a rare problem, but one should be suspicious of a history of a tearing sensation or trauma, with sudden-onset of pain over the lateral epicondyle and forearm. Weakness of grip is profound and, although there is very little published, in our experience this does not settle with time or therapy and the injury is best repaired anatomically with a suture anchor technique.

8.6 Common Flexor Origin: Golfers' Elbow/Medial Epicondylitis

If the tendinopathy arises in the common flexor origin, it is termed medial epicondylitis (ME), or Golfer's elbow. The incidence of medial epicondylitis is approximately five times lower than tennis elbow, although the pathology is the same. As such, the literature is less abundant. The pronator teres tendon is the principal culprit and the provocative test involves resisted pronation with the elbow extended. Some authors suggest that weakness in the flexor pronator muscles predisposes to medial tensile overload. This notion is supported by the high incidence (44%) of ME in patients with C6 and C7 radiculopathy [46]. In addition to the tendon origin pain, a substantial group also experience ulna nerve symptoms. Neurophysiology may not demonstrate entrapment, but neuritis may, nevertheless, cause symptoms. Differential diagnosis again includes elbow instability, intra-articular elbow pathology and pronator syndrome. The principles of management echo those for LE, with an eccentric programme, stretching and activity modification forming the first line of management. Autologous blood injection has shown improvement in symptoms from baseline at 4 weeks and 10 months (Level IV) [47]. Corticosteroid injection again shows improvement at 6 weeks, but not at any further time point and the same concerns exist regarding prolonging the natural history of the disease. If surgery is required for recalcitrant cases and there is ulna neuritis, a cubital tunnel release should be performed in addition to the release procedure. A small series of 15 patients with chronic recalcitrant medial epicondylitis achieved excellent results from open release (11/12 responders at 66 months) [48]. Eleven of 12 returned to work within 8 weeks of surgery and DASH and VAS improved significantly.

8.7 Distal Biceps Pathology

8.7.1 Distal Biceps Tendinopathy

Tendinopathy of the distal biceps tendon is uncommon. Again, a degenerative process is thought to provoke symptom onset [49]. Patients report a pain at the front of the elbow made worse by resisted flexion and supination. Examination will reveal an intact, but painful tendon with pain made worse by resisted supination and flexion. Hook testing may be painful, although it should be negative, as no rupture has occurred. Diagnosis may be made on clinical grounds, but MRI imaging may help to identify those with partial tears and plain films may reveal calcification changes at the tuberosity. Ultrasound can also be used. MRI in a flexed, abducted and supinated (FABS) position optimises the view of the distal biceps tendon (Giuffrè and Moss [50]). As for other tendinopathies around the elbow, eccentric physiotherapy is a first line treatment. Many will be expected to improve, but those with ongoing symptoms may benefit from injection. Ultrasound has been assessed as a guidance-tool for peri-tendinous injection in cadavers and both posterior and anterior approaches were effective [51]. Although corticosteroid injection has shown good results in a small retrospective series [52] at long-term follow-up, concerns remain related to the action of corticosteroid and the pathology of tendinopathy. Recent articles have reported on PRP use in distal biceps tendinopathy. One small study showed that four of six patients enjoyed resolution of symptoms with negative provocation signs by 6 weeks from PRP injection [53]. The remaining two underwent repeat injection, one of whom had a partial tear on MRI. At second follow up, both had improved and provocation signs were negative. Pain and Mayo scores improved significantly and there were no complications. A second, larger study has also suggested benefit from PRP injection [54]. Flexion Abduction Supination (FABS) MRI scan is ordered if the diagnosis is in doubt, or there is a history of trauma (to detect partial injury). Initial treatment comprises an eccentric programme and precipitant avoidance. Those who fail to respond to the exercise programme receive an ultrasound-guided PRP injection. It is rare for a patient to require surgery for distal biceps tendinopathy in the absence of a tear.

8.7.2 Partial Tear

Partial tearing of the distal biceps tendon may occur either after a sudden eccentric loading, as for complete rupture, or it may be the result of a chronic degenerative tendinopathy. In an acute injury, symptoms will be similar to a complete rupture; although on examination, the hook test will be negative and intact tendon palpable. In chronic cases, the symptoms mirror those of tendinopathy. US scans can differentiate partial versus complete tearing with 91% accuracy [55]. MRI scanning is useful in quantifying the degree of tendon rupture, with FABS views recommended (Giuffrè and Moss [50]). In general, a tear of <25% (i.e. half of one muscle belly's tendon) can be managed with rehab, injection or surgical debridement [56]. Some propose that a 50% tear can be tolerated, but it is important to appreciate that the insertion is derived from two muscle belly heads—a 50% tear, therefore, probably represents a complete tear of one head. A symptomatic tear greater than 25–50% should be taken down and repaired formally as for a complete rupture [56]. In experienced hands, a distal biceps bursoscopy can be useful in visualising the damaged tendon and debriding partial injury [56]. For those patients who do not improve with physiotherapy or injection, surgery achieves reliable results in terms of pain relief and return to almost normal flexion and supination strength with a low rate of complications in small case series [57, 58].

8.7.3 Complete Rupture

The classic mechanism for acute distal biceps tendon rupture is a sudden eccentric overloading event. This typically affects the middle-aged male. A history of anabolic steroid use is associated with increased risk of tendon rupture, although these patients fare no worse postoperatively than non-steroid users [59]. Patients report a sudden onset of pain, followed rapidly by bruising and swelling in the ante-cubital fossa. Biomechanical study reveals a 30% reduction in flexion power and a 40% reduction in supination strength after distal biceps tendon rupture. On examination, the inability to hook one's finger around the biceps tendon with the elbow flexed to 90° and the forearm supinated confirms complete rupture [60]. It is important to recognise that the O'Driscoll hook test may be falsely negative in cases where the tendon is torn but the lacertus fibrous remains intact and is tethering the ruptured tendon. In cases where doubt exists regarding degree of injury an urgent ultrasound or 'FABS' MRI can be useful.

While some patients tolerate well the functional loss of a torn distal biceps, most active patients will opt for surgical fixation. Anatomic repair achieves consistently good results [61] and surgical repair has been shown to provide superior outcomes to non-operative management in all measures at 2-year follow-up in a comparative study [62]. The surgical approach used to perform the repair, and the method of fixation seems not to affect significantly the overall outcome. In our practice, we employ a single incision and endobutton bi-cortical fixation [63].

Complications, although rare, include heterotopic ossification, cutaneous or posterior interosseous nerve injury (usually temporary), infection and re-rupture. Active range of motion without resistance can be permitted immediately after surgery, but surgeons employing suture anchors often protect their repair for a few weeks. Resistance training is allowed at 3 months postop. Re-rupture rate is very low at 1.5% [64]. Our institution recently presented a series of cases of symptomatic failure of footprint healing, without frank re-ruptures. All followed suture-anchor fixation and we believe tendon gapping has resulted in failure to achieve on-bone healing. All cases were revised using our standard in-bone endobutton technique. Almost normal functional strength compared to the uninjured side can be expected. Complications, such as heterotopic ossification, increase if surgery is performed more than 2 weeks after the injury so prompt onward referral is recommended.

8.7.4   Irreparable Tendon Injury

Delayed presentation and diagnostic delay can present the surgeon with an injury that may not be directly repairable because the tendon has retracted, scarred and atrophied. These are often referred to as chronic injuries but time alone is not the factor that dictates the ability to repair the tendon. A complete rupture with an intact lacertus fibrosus is likely to be directly repairable even many months after the injury, as the tendon has been held out to length. Although it may be necessary to perform the repair with the elbow joint in a degree of flexion this causes little concern as the biceps muscle will stretch with activity and normal range of motion will be restored. Those with significant tendon retraction and fibrosis require interposition allograft or autograft reconstruction—our preference is allograft tendo-Achilles in a modification of the Mayo clinic's technique [65]. Rehabilitation after allograft reconstruction takes longer (usually 6 months), but patients can still expect good or excellent functional outcome.

8.8   Distal Triceps

Symptomatic pathology of the triceps tendon is uncommon. Weight lifters are more prone to suffering from the condition. If the onset is acute, it is worth excluding an enthesophyte avulsion fracture as the cause of pain with a lateral radiograph and tendon rupture should also be considered. Treatment follows the same principles as for LE and ME, with eccentric exercise being the first-line therapy, leading to PRP injection in recalcitrant cases. We are not aware of any reports of surgery for triceps tendinopathy.

An enthesophyte avulsion fracture describes the pull-off of a small bony spur, with some of the triceps enthesis, from the olecranon. It does not lead to any discontinuity in the triceps tendon and function is not affected.

8.8.1   Triceps Tendon Rupture

Triceps rupture is extremely rare, with only 8 cases from 1014 tendon injuries reported by the Mayo clinic [66]. The tendon is normally avulsed from its insertion on the olecranon process and usually takes with it a fleck of bone (the flake sign) [67]. Patients present with pain, swelling and weakness of active elbow extension (Farrar and Lippert [68]). Metabolic bone disease, steroid injection, rheumatoid arthritis are all associated with increased risk of rupture. Total elbow replacement, particularly revision cases with triceps detachment can also threaten the distal triceps: The Mayo clinic reported ten cases over a 20-year period [69]. Bodybuilders and collision football players are also at greater risk of rupture [70]. The rupture may be either partial or complete, a distinction of importance if one is considering conservative management in partial injuries (Farrar and Lippert [68]). The mechanism is classically a sudden eccentric triceps contraction, with or without a direct blow—a fall onto an outstretched arm is a common mechanism. In cases of complete rupture, there may be a palpable gap just proximal to the tip of the olecranon and loss of active elbow extension. However, the rarity of the injury, pain and swelling may impede initial diagnosis and cases are often missed. MRI and US are useful imaging modalities to confirm and quantify triceps injury [71]. Surgery is recommended for complete ruptures and those cases with more than 50% disruption. The width of the tendon proper is 21 mm in a cadaveric study [72]. In ten professional American football players with partial injury, six returned to full play without surgery [70].

For those that need surgery, Farrar reported success with transosseous suture repair through tunnels drilled into the olecranon [68]. Good results can be expected in acute repair [73], although the Mayo clinic reported a 21% re-rupture rate in their 14 primary repairs. Despite this, in the same study, the long-term strength was 82% of the uninjured side with symmetrical endurance. For two neglected ruptures, with retraction of the muscle, Yazdi performed a V-Y advancement of the triceps tendon and direct repair without the need for turn-down flap or allograft interposition and gained good results [74]. More complex reconstructions, with anconeus rotation, interposition allografts have also been employed [75].

8.9 Conclusion

Tendon injury includes a spectrum of pathology from reactive tendinopathy to chronic tendon rupture. Identification of the stage of pathology is key to providing appropriate treatment. Despite the prevalence of these conditions there is a paucity of good quality literature to guide management and many questions remain un-answered.

Q&A
Q1: Describe the pathological process that leads to tendinopathy.

Tendinopathies are considered to occur as a result of a disruption of normal tissue homeostasis. There is a continuum of pathology from reactive tendinopathy, through tendon disrepair to degenerative tendinopathy. Reactive tendinopathy is readily reversible condition associated with proteoglycan accumulation and oedema. If overload continues there is an increase in matrix production, resulting in both collagen and proteoglycan synthesis known as tendon disrepair. The final stage of degeneration is associated with angiofibroplastic hyperplasia and tenocyte cell death with hypocellular collagen voids. This can weaken the tendon and may lead to tendon rupture.

Q2: What is the best initial treatment for a patient with tennis elbow?

Patients with recent onset symptoms of tennis elbow should be advised to avoid aggravating activities, to take oral analgesia and to consult a physiotherapist. In athletes a reactive tendinopathy can result from overtraining and immediate rest and alternate day isometric exercises are recommended. In more established cases a controlled loading programme is recommended. Steroid injections should be avoided.

Q3: Who is at risk of distal biceps tendon rupture?

The peak incidence of distal biceps rupture is in the fifth decade of life but traumatic avulsion is seen in athletes at a younger age. The risk is higher in contact sports such as rugby. With advancing age a greater proportion of patients report prodromal pain symptoms suggesting that tendopathy may predispose to tendon failure.

Q4: What symptoms and signs should raise a suspicion of distal triceps tendon rupture and how would you investigate further?

Patient will typically report a feeling of tearing at the back of the elbow with loading. The patient is often involved in weight lifting or contact sports activities but certain systemic illnesses are associated including metabolic bone disease and rheumatoid arthritis. There is likely to be weakness of elbow extension but extension against gravity is usually possible due to the intact muscular medial head. A palpable gap may be found on examination and the muscle belly will be high riding in full elbow extension. If the diagnosis is not clear an MRI or ultrasound scan are the investigations of choice.

References

1. Riley G. The pathogenesis of tendinopathy. A molecular perspective. Rheumatology. 2004;43(2):131–42.
2. Nirschl RP. Elbow tendinosis/tennis elbow. Clin Sports Med. 1992;11(4):851–70.
3. Cook JL, Purdam CR. Is tendon pathology a continuum? A pathology model to explain the clinical presentation of load-induced tendinopathy. Br J Sports Med. 2009;43(6):409–16.
4. Tallon C, Coleman BD, Khan KM, Maffulli N. Outcome of surgery for chronic Achilles tendinopathy: a critical review. Am J Sports Med. 2001;29(3):315–20.
5. Rio E, Moseley L, Purdam C, Samiric T, Kidgell D, Pearce AJ, Jaberzadeh S, Cook J. The pain of tendinopathy: physiological or pathophysiological? Sports Med. 2014;44(1):9–23.
6. Alfredson H, Thorsen K, Lorentzon R. In situ microdialysis in tendon tissue: high levels of glutamate, but not prostaglandin E2 in chronic Achilles tendon pain. Knee Surg Sports Traumatol. 1999;7:378–81.
7. Coombes BK, Bisset L, Vicenzino B. Efficacy and safety of corticosteroid injections and other injections for management of tendinopathy: a systematic review of randomised controlled trials. Lancet. 2010;376(9754):1751–67.

8. Buchbinder R, Green SE, Struijs PA. Tennis elbow. BMJ Clin Evid. 2008;2008.

9. Chiang HC, Ko YC, Chen SS, Yu HS, Wu TN, Chang PY. Prevalence of shoulder and upper-limb disorders among workers in the fish-processing industry. Scand J Work Environ Health. 1993;19:126–31.

10. Greenfield C, Webster V. Chronic lateral epicondylitis: survey of current practice in the outpatient departments in scotland. Physiotherapy. 2002;88(10):578–94.

11. Nirschl RP. The etiology and treatment of tennis elbow. J Sports Med. 1974;2(6):308–23.

12. Assendelft WJ, Hay EM, Adshead R, Bouter LM. Corticosteroid injections for lateral epicondylitis: a systematic overview. Br J Gen Pract. 1996;46(405):209–16.

13. Bisset L, Beller E, Jull G, Brooks P, Darnell R, Vicenzino B. Mobilisation with movement and exercise, corticosteroid injection, or wait and see for tennis elbow: randomised trial. BMJ. 2006;333(7575):939.

14. Smidt N, Van Der Windt DA, Assendelft WJ, Devillé WL, Korthals-de Bos IB, Bouter LM. Corticosteroid injections, physiotherapy, or a wait-and-see policy for lateral epicondylitis: a randomised controlled trial. Lancet. 2002;359(9307):657–62.

15. Walton MJ, Mackie K, Fallon M, Butler R, Breidahl W, Zheng MH, Wang A. The reliability and validity of magnetic resonance imaging in the assessment of chronic lateral epicondylitis. J Hand Surg. 2011;36(3):475–9.

16. Latham SK, Smith TO. The diagnostic test accuracy of ultrasound for the detection of lateral epicondylitis: a systematic review and meta-analysis. Orthopaed Traumatol Surg Res. 2014;100(3):281 6.

17. Hudak PL, Cole DC, Haines AT. Understanding prognosis to improve rehabilitation: the example of lateral elbow pain. Arch Phys Med Rehabil. 1996;77(6):586–93.

18. Jones VA. Physiotherapy in the management of tennis elbow: a review. Should Elb. 2009;1(2):108–13.

19. Alfredson H, Pietilä T, Jonsson P, Lorentzon R. Heavy-load eccentric calf muscle training for the treatment of chronic Achilles tendinosis. Am J Sports Med. 1998;26(3):360–6.

20. Öhberg L, Alfredson H. Effects on neovascularisation behind the good results with eccentric training in chronic mid-portion Achilles tendinosis? Knee Surg Sports Traumatol Arthrosc. 2004;12(5):465–70.

21. Svernlöv B, Adolfsson L. Non-operative treatment regime including eccentric training for lateral humeral epicondylalgia. Scand J Med Sci Sports. 2001;11(6):328–34.

22. Crosier J, Foidart-Desalle M, Godon B, Crielaard J-M. Treatment of recurrent tendinitis by isokinetic eccentric exercises. Isokinet Exerc Sci. 2001;9:133–41.

23. Cullinane FL, Boocock MG, Trevelyan FC. Is eccentric exercise an effective treatment for lateral epicondylitis? A systematic review. Clin Rehabil. 2014;28(1):3–19.

24. Pienimäki T, Karinen P, Kemilä T, Koivukangas P, Vanharanta H. Long-term follow-up of conservatively treated chronic tennis elbow patients. A prospective and retrospective analysis. Scand J Rehabil Med. 1998;30(3):159–66.

25. Hoogvliet P, Randsdorp MS, Dingemanse R, Koes BW, Huisstede BM. Does effectiveness of exercise therapy and mobilisation techniques offer guidance for the treatment of lateral and medial epicondylitis? A systematic review. Br J Sports Med. 2013;47(17):1112–9.

26. Jensen B, Bliddal H, Danneskiold-Samsøe B. Comparison of two different treatments of lateral humeral epicondylitis – "tennis elbow". A randomized controlled trial. Ugeskr Laeger. 2001;163(10):1427–31.

27. Wuori JL, Overend TJ, Kramer JF, MacDermid J. Strength and pain measures associated with lateral epicondylitis bracing. Arch Phys Med Rehabil. 1998;79(7):832–7.

28. Garg R, Adamson GJ, Dawson PA, Shankwiler JA, Pink MM. A prospective randomized study comparing a forearm strap brace versus a wrist splint for the treatment of lateral epicondylitis. J Shoulder Elb Surg. 2010;19(4):508–12.

29. Dingemanse R, Randsdorp M, Koes BW, Huisstede BM. Evidence for the effectiveness of electrophysical modalities for treatment of medial and lateral epicondylitis: a systematic review. Br J Sports Med. 2014;48(12):957–65.

30. Bisset L, Paungmali A, Vicenzino B, Beller E. A systematic review and meta-analysis of clinical trials on physical interventions for lateral epicondylalgia. Br J Sports Med. 2005;39(7):411–22.

31. Haake M, Böddeker I, Decker T, Buch M, Vogel M, Labek G, Maier M, Loew M, Maier-Boerries O, Fischer J, Betthäuser A. Side-effects of extracorporeal shock wave therapy (ESWT) in the treatment of tennis elbow. Arch Orthop Trauma Surg. 2002;122(4):222–8.

32. Speed CA, Nichols D, Richards C, Humphreys H, Wies JT, Burnet S, Hazleman BL. Extracorporeal shock wave therapy for lateral epicondylitis—a double blind randomized controlled trial. J Orthop Res. 2002;20(5):895–8.

33. Buchbinder R, Green SE, Youd JM, Assendelft WJ, Barnsley L, Smidt N. Shock wave therapy for lateral elbow pain. Cochrane Database Syst Rev. 2009;4:CD003524.

34. Olaussen M, Holmedal O, Lindbaek M, Brage S, Solvang H. Treating lateral epicondylitis with corticosteroid injections or non-electrotherapeutical physiotherapy: a systematic review. BMJ Open. 2013;3(10):e003564.

35. Coombes BK, Bisset L, Brooks P, Khan A, Vicenzino B. Effect of corticosteroid injection, physiotherapy, or both on clinical outcomes in patients with unilateral lateral epicondylalgia: a randomized controlled trial. JAMA. 2013;309(5):461–9.

36. Hayton MJ, Santini AJ, Hughes PJ, Frostick SP, Trail IA, Stanley JK. Botulinum toxin injection in the treatment of tennis elbow: a double-blind, randomized, controlled, pilot study. JBJS. 2005;87(3):503–7.

37. Lin YC, Tu YK, Chen SS, Lin IL, Chen SC, Guo HR. Comparison between botulinum toxin and corticosteroid injection in the treatment of acute and subacute tennis elbow: a prospective, randomized, double-blind, active drug-controlled pilot study. Am J Phys Med Rehabil. 2010;89(8):653–9.

38. Kalichman L, Bannuru RR, Severin M, Harvey W. Injection of botulinum toxin for treatment of chronic lateral epicondylitis: systematic review and meta-analysis. Semin Arthritis Rheumat. 2011;40(6):532–8.

39. Petrella RJ, Cogliano A, Decaria J, Mohamed N, Lee R. Management of tennis elbow with sodium hyaluronate periarticular injections. BMC Sports Sci Med Rehabil. 2010;2(1):4.

40. Moraes VY, Lenza M, Tamaoki MJ, Faloppa F, Belloti JC. Platelet-rich therapies for musculoskeletal soft tissue injuries. Cochrane Database Syst Rev. 2014;4.

41. Mishra AK, Skrepnik NV, Edwards SG, Jones GL, Sampson S, Vermillion DA, Ramsey ML, Karli DC, Rettig AC. Efficacy of platelet-rich plasma for chronic tennis elbow: a double-blind, prospective, multicenter, randomized controlled trial of 230 patients. Am J Sports Med. 2014;42(2):463–71.

42. Thanasas C, Papadimitriou G, Charalambidis C, Paraskevopoulos I, Papanikolaou A. Platelet-rich plasma versus autologous whole blood for the treatment of chronic lateral elbow epicondylitis: a randomized controlled clinical trial. Am J Sports Med. 2011;39(10):2130–4.

43. Creaney L, Wallace A, Curtis M, Connell D. Growth factor-based therapies provide additional benefit beyond physical therapy in resistant elbow tendinopathy: a prospective, single-blind, randomised trial of autologous blood injections versus platelet-rich plasma injections. Br J Sports Med. 2011;45(12):966–71.

44. Wang A, Breidahl W, Mackie KE, Lin Z, Qin A, Chen J, Zheng MH. Autologous tenocyte injection for the treatment of severe, chronic resistant lateral epicondylitis: a pilot study. Am J Sports Med. 2013;41(12):2925–32.

45. Wang A, Mackie K, Breidahl W, Wang T, Zheng MH. Evidence for the durability of autologous tenocyte injection for treatment of chronic resistant lateral epicondylitis: mean 4.5-year clinical follow-up. Am J Sports Med. 2015;43(7):1775–83.

46. Lee A, Lee-Robinson A. Evaluating concomitant lateral epicondylitis and cervical radiculopathy: a correlation was found, suggesting comanagement of the disorders. J Musculoskel Med. 2010;27(3):111.

47. Suresh SP, Ali KE, Jones H, Connell DA. Medial epicondylitis: is ultrasound guided autologous blood injection an effective treatment? Br J Sports Med. 2006;40(11):935–9.

48. Shahid M, Wu F, Deshmukh SC. Operative treatment improves patient function in recalcitrant

medial epicondylitis. Ann Roy Coll Surgeons Engl. 2013;95(7):486–8.

49. Bachoura A, Sasaki K, Kamineni S. Analysis of age-related degenerative changes of the biceps brachii distal footprint. J Surg Orthop Adv. 2013;22(4):304–9.

50. Giuffre BM, Moss MJ. Optimal positioning for MRI of the distal biceps brachii tendon: flexed abducted supinated view. Am J Roentgenol. 2004;182(4):944–6.

51. Sellon JL, Wempe MK, Smith J. Sonographically guided distal biceps tendon injections: techniques and validation. J Ultrasound Med. 2014;33(8):1461–74.

52. Maree MN, Vrettos BC, Roche SJ, Osch GV. Distal biceps tendinopathy: conservative treatment. Should Elb. 2011;3(2):104–8.

53. Barker SL, Bell SN, Connell D, Coghlan JA. Ultrasound-guided platelet-rich plasma injection for distal biceps tendinopathy. Should Elb. 2015;7(2):110–4.

54. Sanli I, Morgan B, van Tilborg F, Funk L, Gosens T. Single injection of platelet-rich plasma (PRP) for the treatment of refractory distal biceps tendonitis: long-term results of a prospective multicenter cohort study. Knee Surg Sports Traumatol Arthrosc. 2016;24(7):2308–12.

55. Lobo LD, Fessell DP, Miller BS, Kelly A, Lee JY, Brandon C, Jacobson JA. The role of sonography in differentiating full versus partial distal biceps tendon tears: correlation with surgical findings. Am J Roentgenol. 2013;200(1):158–62.

56. Bain GI, Johnson LJ, Turner PC. Treatment of partial distal biceps tendon tears. Sports Med Arthrosc Rev. 2008;16(3):154–61.

57. Frazier MS, Boardman MJ, Westland M, Imbriglia JE. Surgical treatment of partial distal biceps tendon ruptures. J Hand Surg. 2010;35(7):1111–4.

58. Vardakas DG, Musgrave DS, Varitimidis SE, Goebel F, Sotereanos DG. Partial rupture of the distal biceps tendon. J Shoulder Elb Surg. 2001;10(4):377–9.

59. Pagonis T, Givissis P, Ditsios K, Pagonis A, Petsatodis G, Christodoulou A. The effect of steroid-abuse on anatomic reinsertion of ruptured distal biceps brachii tendon. Injury. 2011;42(11):1307–12.

60. O'Driscoll SW, Goncalves LB, Dietz P. The hook test for distal biceps tendon avulsion. Am J Sports Med. 2007;35(11):1865–9.

61. Sarda P, Qaddori A, Nauschutz F, Boulton L, Nanda R, Bayliss N. Distal biceps tendon rupture: current concepts. Injury. 2013;44(4):417–20.

62. Chillemi C, Marinelli M, De Cupis V. Rupture of the distal biceps brachii tendon: conservative treatment versus anatomic reinsertion—clinical and radiological evaluation after 2 years. Arch Orthop Trauma Surg. 2007;127(8):705–8.

63. Bain GI, Prem H, Heptinstall RJ, Verhellen R, Paix D. Repair of distal biceps tendon rupture: A new technique using the endobutton. J Shoulder Elb Surg. 2000;9(2):120–6. ISSN 1058-2746, https://doi.org/10.1067/2000.102581 (http://www.sciencedirect.com/science/article/pii/S1058274600900405).

64. Hinchey JW, Aronowitz JG, Sanchez-Sotelo J, Morrey BF. Re-rupture rate of primarily repaired distal biceps tendon injuries. J Shoulder Elb Surg. 2014;23(6):850–4.

65. Phadnis J, Flannery O, Watts AC. Distal biceps reconstruction using an Achilles tendon allograft, transosseous EndoButton, and Pulvertaft weave with tendon wrap technique for retracted, irreparable distal biceps ruptures. J Shoulder Elb Surg. 2016;25(6):1013–9.

66. Anzel SH, Covey KW, Weiner AD, Lipscomb PR. Disruption of muscles and tendons: an analysis of 1,014 cases. Surgery. 1959;45(3):406–14.

67. Pina A, Garcia I, Sabater M. Traumatic avulsion of the triceps brachii. J Orthop Trauma. 2002;16(4):273–6.

68. Farrar EL III, Lippert FG III. Avulsion of the triceps tendon. Clin Orthopaed Relat Res (1976–2007). 1981;161:242–6.

69. Van Riet RP, Morrey BF, Ho E, O'Driscoll SW. Surgical treatment of distal triceps ruptures. JBJS. 2003;85(10):1961–7.

70. Mair SD, Isbell WM, Gill TJ, Schlegel TF, Hawkins RJ. Triceps tendon ruptures in professional football players. Am J Sports Med. 2004;32(2):431–4.

71. Tagliafico A, Gandolfo N, Michaud J, Perez MM, Palmieri F, Martinoli C. Ultrasound demonstration of distal triceps tendon tears. Eur J Radiol. 2012;81(6):1207–10.

72. Keener JD, Chafik D, Kim HM, Galatz LM, Yamaguchi K. Insertional anatomy of the triceps brachii tendon. J Shoulder Elb Surg. 2010;19(3):399–405.

73. Holleb PD, Bach BR. Triceps brachii injuries. Sports Med. 1990;10(4):273–6.

74. Yazdi HR, Qomashi I, Ghorban HM. Neglected triceps tendon avulsion: case report, literature review, and a new repair method. Am J Orthop. 2012;41(7):E96–9.

75. Sanchez-Sotelo J, Morrey BF. Surgical techniques for reconstruction of chronic insufficiency of the triceps: rotation flap using anconeus and tendo achillis allograft. J Bone Joint Surg Br. 2002;84(8):1116–20.

Myofascial Syndromes

9

Philip Holland and Adam C. Watts

Contents

Key Learning Points

1. Exertional compartment syndrome of the forearm is initially treated with activity modification.
2. Surgery has good results for exertional compartment syndrome of the forearm resistant to activity modification.
3. Forearm splints are common amongst pommel horse gymnasts.
4. The treatment of forearm splints is activity modification.
5. There is no single diagnostic investigation for forearm splints or exertional compartment syndrome of the forearm.

P. Holland · A. C. Watts (✉)
Wrightington Hospital Upper Limb Unit, Wigan, UK
e-mail: adam.watts@elbowdoc.co.uk

9.1 Exertional Compartment Syndrome of the Forearm (Arm Pump)

9.1.1 Introduction

Chronic exertional compartment syndrome of the forearm (CECSf) is a clinical syndrome of forearm pain on exercise. The typical exercises that cause CECSf are constant forceful gripping. CECSf is the upper limb equivalent of the more common form of exertional compartment syndrome that affects the lower leg. It is colloquially known amongst athletes as "arm pump".

CECSf occurs when the compartment pressure is higher than the capillary perfusion pressure. Any one or more of the four forearm

A. C. Watts et al. (eds.), *Sports Injuries of the Elbow*, https://doi.org/10.1007/978-3-030-52379-4_9

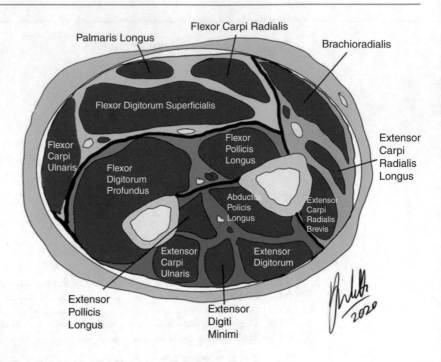

Fig. 9.1 Forearm myofascial compartments (note—all compartments can be involved)

compartments can be involved (Fig. 9.1). Notably, CECSf does not occur every time the compartment pressure is higher than the capillary perfusion pressure. It is likely that there are other environmental and genetic factors that determine if an athlete experiences symptoms or not.

9.1.2 Pathophysiology

During exercise the forearm muscles produce lactic acid that stimulates an increase in blood flow. The muscles are already often large in an athlete and the increase in blood flow further increases the volume of the forearm contents. The fascial compartments have a fixed volume and so the pressure within the forearm increases. The increase in pressure compromises venous return because the veins, which are low pressure, are occluded before the arteries, which are higher pressure. This results in more blood flowing into the forearm than out of the forearm further increasing the forearm pressure. This positive feedback loop is outlined in Fig. 9.2.

The pain caused by CECSf is most likely caused by a combination of the high forearm

pressure itself and the lactic acid build up in the muscles caused by the inadequate blood flow.

It is not known why some athletes suffer with CECSf while others do not. It is more common in young men in who naturally have greater muscle bulk. It has been speculated that some individuals may have a genetic predisposition to CECSf. This is supported by several case reports of bilateral CECSf; case reports of exertional compartment syndrome affecting different anatomical areas and a case report of family members having exertional compartment syndrome [1–5]. Anecdotally, it has been reported that the fascia in patients with CECSf is thicker than normally encountered [6]. Another, equally plausible, explanation as to why some athletes get CECSf while others do not, is that previous injury can cause muscle contusion, swelling and scaring. This could increase the volume of the forearm contents and reduce the ability of the fascial compartments to expand.

The sports that cause CECSf are those that involve constant forceful gripping with little rest time where the compartment pressure can drop below the capillary perfusion pressure. Intermittent or less forceful grips promote venous return and may be protective of CECSf.

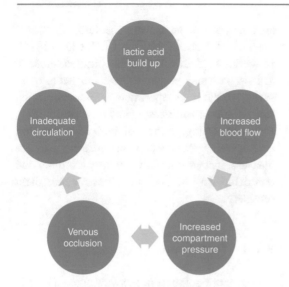

Fig. 9.2 Positive feedback loop causing CECSf

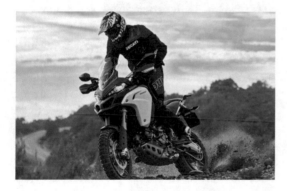

Fig. 9.3 Enduro motorcyclist

Motocross and motorcycle racing are particularly high risk sports because of the combination of constant grip, twisting of the throttle and shocks through the arms. Up to half of enduro motorcyclist riders experience forearm pain after riding (Fig. 9.3) [7]. Other high-risk sports include kayaking, rock climbing and weight lifting (Table 9.1).

9.1.3 Diagnosis

Athletes with CECSf present with forearm pain when they do specific activities. The pain resolves after a period of rest, however, it can persist for

Table 9.1 Sports associated with CECSf and interventions to reduce the risk

Associated activities	Interventions
Climbing	Chalk hands adequately Push up with legs during climbs in preference to pulling up with arms
Gymnastics	Chalk hands adequately High quality hand guard
Hockey	Use a vibration dampening hockey stick High quality grips
Kayaking	Cranked paddle to align forces with the forearm Wax paddle grip to increase friction Ergonomic paddle cross section to facilitate grip
Motocross	Ensure optimal front suspension to reduce shock transmission Ensure optimal bike set up to enable grip from legs
Rowing	Alternate between a strong "drive grip" during the stroke and a weaker "recovery grip" during the feather
Tennis	High quality racket grip Shock absorbers
Waterskiing	High quality handle Consider using a rope with more stretch Change grip position
Weight training	Change grip position High quality gloves
Wheelchair sports	Consider using gloves High quality wheel grip

beyond 12 h. The main concern to athletes is usually a "dead arm" that prevents participation in sport and not the persistent pain [8]. The athlete may also experience numbness in the hand, clumsiness, a loss of muscle strength and cramp. The differential diagnosis includes peripheral nerve entrapment neuropathies, forearm tendinopathies and limb ischemia (Table 9.2).

Clinical examination is usually unremarkable. When the athlete is symptomatic the forearm compartments will be tight to palpate but this is an unreliable sign [8]. An increase in forearm circumference may also be found. Radiographs, ultrasound scans and resting MRI scans are often normal in CECSf but can be useful to exclude other conditions.

Sequential MRI scans immediately after the onset of symptoms and then every 5 min for

Table 9.2 Causes of forearm pain in athletes

Tendinopathies
Golfers elbow
Tennis elbow
Intersection syndrome
De Quervains tenosynovitis
FCR Tendonitis
Compression Neuropathies
Carpal tunnel syndrome
Cubital tunnel syndrome
Radial tunnel syndrome
Pronator syndrome
Radiculopathy
Vascular
Limb ischemia
Thoracic outlet syndrome
Other
Tumours
Infections
Stress fractures
Ganglions

15 min during recovery can be helpful. This can show an area of high signal on the T2 sequence that resolves with resolution of the symptoms [9].

A needle electromyogram (EMG) may show denervation secondary to the increased compartment pressure. Some studies have identified EMG changes that they cannot attribute to cause other than the CECSf [9]. Nevertheless, a normal needle EMG does not exclude CECSf and so this invasive painful investigation is not recommended routinely. Surface nerve conduction studies have not been shown to be affected by CECSf [9].

There is no consensus as to what the normal compartment pressure measurements of the forearm are [10]. It is generally considered that a forearm pressure >10 mmHg at rest or >20 mmHg on exertion is supportive of CECSf [11]. However, lower pressures than this do not exclude CECSf and higher pressures than this can be normal. Compartment pressures as high as 39 mmHg have been recorded in normal forearms and following a surgical fasciectomy forearm compartment pressures that have dropped only to 104 mmHg have had a successful outcome [10].

Measuring changes in compartment pressures with serial measurements has been suggested as an alternative to measuring absolute values as a potential diagnostic tool for CECSf [1, 12–14]. However, to date this has had limited success. This in part may be due to inaccuracies in measuring forearm compartment pressures, which can be due to differences in probe positioning, limb positioning, degree of muscle contraction and operator expertise. Compartment pressure measurements are invasive, time consuming and unreliable so we do not recommend them routinely.

9.1.4 Treatment

Unlike acute compartment syndrome, CECSf is self-limiting; upon the cessation of sustained forceful gripping the symptoms resolve. Athletes often suffer with recurrent symptoms every time they participate in sport. The symptoms can become severe enough to prevent the participation in sport; early intervention may prevent this.

Activity modification is the mainstay of treatment. Athletes can often incorporate periods of grip relaxation during sport even if this is only for a short period of time. Selling this concept to an athlete can be difficult. In some sports such as motocross the athlete will be aware that a period of grip relaxation may have an immediate short term detrimental effect on performance. When discussing this it is important to stress that grip relaxation may improve endurance and so improve overall performance. Some sports, such as rowing, alternate between a "drive grip" and "recovery grip". Emphasising the endurance benefits of utilising the recovery grip better can improve endurance with no detrimental effect on performance.

The strength of the grip required for sport can be reduced by optimising the ergonomics of the object they are gripping. An example of this is in kayakers where often a round paddle shaft is used. This requires a tight grip to prevent it slipping. An oval paddle shaft reduces the grip pressure required.

Some sports have different techniques that can be used for gripping. An example of this is that water-skiers can choose to hold the handle in different ways. This includes one palm up with one palm down, both palms down or both palms up. Athletes may be reluctant to change their grip, but if doing so for a period of time allows them to train for longer, they may be receptive to this. Some other sport specific adaptations are suggested in Table 9.1.

It is unlikely that athletes who have intolerable symptoms despite activity modification will have any improvement in their symptoms over time [1]. A surgical forearm fasciotomy or partial fasciectomy is recommended for these patients. A fasciectomy has the theoretical advantage of reducing the risk of the fascia healing in the same place leaving the compartment volume unchanged. Both fasciotomies and fasciectomies have been shown to be successful in managing persistent symptoms [5, 6, 8].

Following surgery patients can be back to sport as early as 4 weeks post-operatively. Most patients have some long-term improvement in their symptoms [5, 6, 8]. Failure to improve is likely to be either because the fasciotomy has scarred, reforming a tight compartment, or the diagnosis was incorrect. The reported complications are haematoma formation, cutaneous nerve injury and widening of the scar over time [5, 6].

9.2 Forearm Splints (Pommel Arm)

9.2.1 Introduction

Forearm splints are pain experienced in the forearm, often during repeated forceful eccentric muscle contraction. The exact cause is poorly understood but they are thought to be the counterpart to shin splints in the lower limb. Gymnasts using the pommel horse are the most commonly affected athletes, which has led to the colloquial term "pommel arm".

9.2.2 Pathophysiology

The pathophysiology of forearm splints is unknown. It has been suggested that forceful eccentric muscle contractions stress the muscles attached to the radius, ulna and interosseous membrane [15]. It is thought this may lead to periostitis although this has not been proven histologically. Flexor digitorum profundus has a large attachment to the ulna, and flexor pollicis longus has a large attachment to the radius and so these muscles are most likely the cause of forearm splints (Fig. 9.4).

Deep tissue massage has been reported to improve shin splints more quickly than no treatment [16]. Advocates of this treatment suggest a fascial distortion model, whereby connections between fascial layers exist that lead to abnormal traction and pain. They report deep massage breaks these down. In forearm splints athletes often use isotonic exercises with the hand in a rice bucket that may have a similar effect on any abnormal fascial connections (Fig. 9.5). Although unproven the fascia distortion model does provide an alternative hypothesis as to the pathology of forearm splints.

It is important to note that forearm splints are not caused by stress fractures, CECSf or traumatic periostitis. If these conditions are identified, then they should be treated before diagnosis of forearm splints is made.

9.2.3 Diagnosis

Athletes with forearm splints complain of a sharp, localised, sudden onset of pain in the forearm during repetitive forceful eccentric loading. The athlete may report that it feels like the bone will break. This classically occurs in gymnasts doing turns on a pommel horse or when performing a planche (Fig. 9.6).

The pain can be anywhere in the forearm and is often felt on the dorsal or ulnar sides. It typically resolves quickly on stopping exercise. Examination may identify tender areas but is otherwise unremarkable.

Radiographs, MRI scans and isotope bone scans can all show abnormalities in the presence of periostitis [15]. However, periostitis can have different causes including stress fractures, tumours, infections and trauma. It is, therefore,

Fig. 9.4 Muscle attachments in forearm

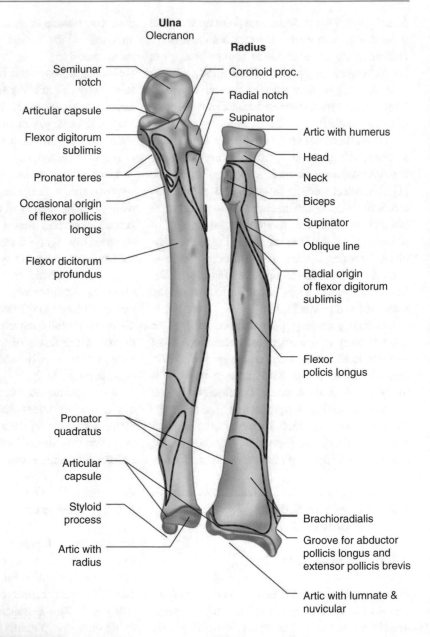

important to interpret imaging in context with the clinical history. In the investigation of shin splints T2-weighted MRI scans have shown periosteal high signal in up to 40% of patients [17]. Assuming a similar pathology, MRI scans may be a useful in diagnosing forearm splints.

9.2.4   Treatment

The prevention of forearm splints is important for high-risk athletes, particularly gymnasts.

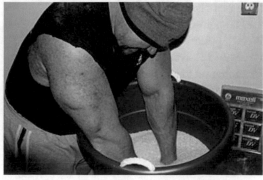

Fig. 9.5   Rice bucket exercises (t-nation.com)

Fig. 9.6 Planche
(Wikipedia.org)

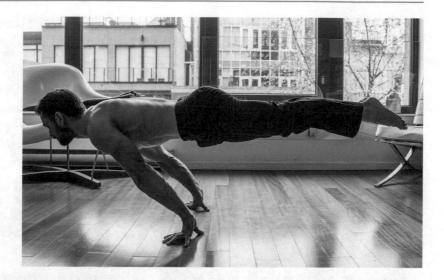

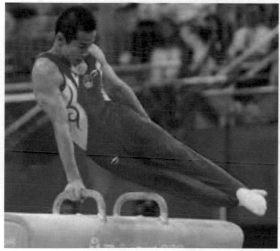

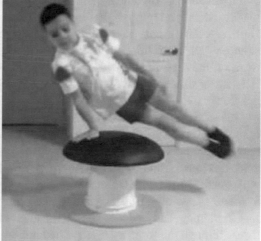

Fig. 9.7 Pommel horse and training mushroom

Forearm splints have been widely attributed to training at a level that is too high for the condition of the wrists and forearms. It is important to work on conditioning the wrists and forearms as much as possible. One way to condition the wrists is for athletes to transition from the training mushroom to the pommel horse early on in their career (Fig. 9.7). The pommel horse strengthens the wrist and forearm in a more functional way than the training mushroom. When training on the pommel horse, the intensity should be graduated and appropriate to the athlete. A thorough warm up and cool down should always be used.

When an athlete suffers with forearm splints the initial treatment involves a period of relative rest by activity modification. Analgesics and NSAIDs can also be used. Deep tissue massage may also be tried and advocates suggest this may break down adhesions between the fascial compartments in the forearm [16]. There is also week evidence that extracorporeal shockwave therapy may shorten the duration of shin splints, but there are no reports of its use in the upper limb [18]. Once the forearm splints have resolved, if the athlete returns to their previous activity the forearm splints are likely to return. Some permanent activity modification should be considered.

Fig. 9.8 Pommel horse rotations

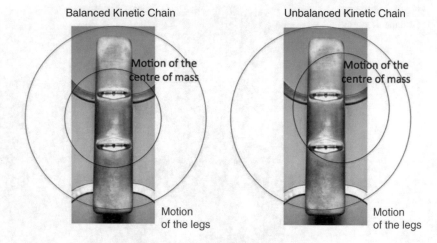

Balanced Kinetic Chain

Motion of the centre of mass

Motion of the legs

Unbalanced Kinetic Chain

Motion of the centre of mass

Motion of the legs

When returning to training, the initial rehabilitation should involve less forceful eccentric loading than precipitated the forearm splints. High repetitions can be used to optimise the strength gain from this. These exercises should work on the long flexors and extensors particularly flexor digitorum profundus and flexor pollicis longus.

One of the most important activity modifications is training optimisation. When training on the pommel horse every turn should be considered precious. Athletes should perform fewer high-quality turns; with the coach watching each turn and a specific goal for each turn. This optimises training and reduces the summation of forces through the forearm. A suggested training routine could be to have a maximum of three attempts at any specific sequence and not to do more than 20 circles in a set.

The entire kinetic chain should be considered when treating a gymnast with forearm splints. Whilst using the pommel horse, a gymnast's kinetic chain has two rotations. The first is the rotation of the legs around the body. The second is the rotation of the bodies centre of mass (Fig. 9.8).

Asymmetrical rotation of the centre of mass increases the forces placed through the forearms and wrists [19]. As well as rotational movements, whilst using the pommel horse, gymnasts also have a vertical motion. Minimising this and keeping it smooth reduces the forces through the forearms.

Wrist supports are widely used by gymnasts to prevent forearm splints although it is preferable, when possible, to condition the forearms sufficiently to avoid this.

Q&A

Q—What is the most useful investigation for CECS?

A—Sequential MRI scans every performed every 5 min from the onset of symptoms, brought about by forearm exertion exercises such as squeezing a sphygmometer bulb, can show oedema changes within the muscle. Forearm compartment pressure monitoring is invasive and there is no true "cut off" for diagnosis.

Q—What non-surgical adaptations might a motocross rider do to prevent CECSf?

A—Ensure optimal set up to enable grip from legs.

Ensure suspension optimally set up.

Relax grip when safe while riding.

Q—What are the surgical options to treat CECSf?

A—Fasciotomy.

Partial fasciectomy.

Q—What athlete is at most risk from forearm splints?

A—Pommel horse gymnast.

Q—Are forearm splints and periostitis the same condition?

A—No. Forearm splints are thought to be one of several causes of periostitis.

References

1. Garcia Mata S, Hidalgo Ovejero A, Martinez Grande M. Bilateral, chronic exertional compartment syndrome of the forearm in two brothers. Clin J Sport Med. 1999;9:91–9.
2. Hider SL, Hilton RC, Hutchinson C. Chronic exertional compartment syndrome as a cause of bilateral forearm pain. Arthritis Rheum. 2002;46:2245–6.
3. Pedowitz RA, Toutounghi FM. Chronic exertional compartment syndrome of the forearm flexor muscles. J Hand Surg Am. 1988;13:694–6.
4. Piasecki DP, Meyer D, Bach BR. Exertional compartment syndrome of the forearm in an elite flatwater sprint kayaker. Am J Sports Med. 2008;36: 2222–5.
5. Zandi H, Bell S. Results of compartment decompression in chronic forearm compartment syndrome: six case presentations. Br J Sports Med. 2005;39:35.
6. Brown JS, Wheeler KT, Boyd MR, Barnes MR, Allen MJ. Chronic exertional compartment syndrome of the forearm: a case series of 12 patients treated with fasciotomy. J Hand Surg Eur Vol. 2011;36:413–9.
7. Sabeti-Aschraf M, Serek M, Pachtner T, Auner K, Machinek M, Geisler M, Goll A. The Enduro motorcyclist's wrist and other overuse injuries in competitive Enduro motorcyclists: a prospective study. Scand J Med Sci Sports. 2008;18:582–90.
8. Winkes MB, Luiten EJT, van Zoest WJF, Sala HA, Hoogeveen AR, Scheltinga MR. Long-term results of surgical decompression of chronic exertional compartment syndrome of the forearm in motocross racers. Am J Med. 2012;40:452–8.
9. Amendola A, Rorabeck CH, Vellett D, Vezina W, Rutt B, Nott L. The use of magnetic resonance imaging in exertional compartment syndromes. Am J Sports Med. 1990;18(1):29–34.
10. Schoeffl V, Klee S, Strecker W. Evaluation of physiological standard pressures of the forearm flexor muscles during sport specific ergometry in sport climbers. Br J Sports Med. 2004;38:422–5.
11. Rydholm U, Brun A, Ekelund L, Rydholm A. Chronic compartment syndrome in the tensor fasciae lata muscle. Clin Orthoped Relat Res. 1983;177:169.
12. Goubier JN, Saillant G. Chronic compartment syndrome of the forearm in competitive motor cyclists: a report of two cases. Br J Sports Med. 2003;37:452–3.
13. Kutz JE, Singer R, Lindsay M. Chronic exertional compartment syndrome of the forearm: a case report. J Hand Surg Am. 1985;10:302–4.
14. Soderberg TA. Bilateral chronic compartment syndrome in the forearm and the hand. J Bone Joint Surg Br. 1996;78:780–2.
15. Wadwhwa SS, Mansberg R, Fernandes VB, Qasim S. Forearm splints seen on bone scan in a weightlifter. Clin Nucl Med. 1997;22(10):711–2.
16. Schultz C, Finze S, Bader R, Lison A. Treatment of medial tibial stress syndrome according to the fascial distortion model: a prospective case control study. Scientific World J. 2014;2014:1–6.
17. Moen MH, Schmikli SL, Weir A, Steeneken V, Stapper G, de Slegte R, Tol JL, Backx FJ. A prospective study on MRI findings and prognostic factors in athletes with MTSS. Scand J Med Sci Sports. 2014;24(1):204–10.
18. Moen MH, Rayer S, Schipper M, Schmikli S, Weir A, Tol JL, Backx FJ. Shockwave treatment for medial tibial stress syndrome in athletes; a prospective controlled study. Br J Sports Med. 2012;46(4):253–7.
19. Fujihara T, Fuchimoto T, Gervais P. Biomechanical analysis of circles on pommel horse. Sports Biomech. 2009;8(1):22–38.

Rehabilitation

10

Jill L. Thomas and Val Jones

Contents

Key Learning Points

- An understanding of the key components of elbow rehabilitation will optimise outcomes and return to sport.
- Early overhead mobilisation is key to prevent stiffness.
- A comprehensive elbow rehabilitation programme should include isometrics, the full kinetic chain and plyometrics.

- Interval programmes should be included in a return to sports programme.

10.1 Introduction

Over recent decades there has been a sharp rise in the number of participants in sport. Injuries to the elbow during sport, such as fracture, dislocation or tendon rupture, can be the result of a single traumatic event. However, most injuries can be attributed to chronic overuse. Sports that are prone to elbow injuries involve those with extensive use of the arm in throwing, e.g. bowling, javelin; those in which the arm is used as a lever

J. L. Thomas (✉)
Wrightington Upper Limb Unit, Wrightington, UK

V. Jones
Sheffield Shoulder and Elbow Unit, Sheffield, UK

Table 10.1 Commonly encountered elbow injuries [5]

Commonly encountered injuries
Lateral ulnar collateral ligament and medial collateral ligament tears
Ulnar nerve lesions
Flexor pronator sprain, tear or tendinopathy
Medial epicondyle apophysitis or avulsion
Lateral epicondylar tendinopathy
Olecranon osteophytes
Olecranon stress fractures
Osteochondritis dissecans
Loose bodies
Distal biceps tendon rupture

for swinging or hitting e.g. tennis, golf and racquetball; and those where the arm is turned into a weight bearing joint e.g. gymnastics and weightlifting. In addition, the elbow can be injured in sport when used to block fired shots such as in rugby, volleyball or goalkeeping in football. Up to 30% of participants engaged in activities such as throwing, bowling, tennis, swimming and volleyball complain of elbow problems [1–4]. The most common athletic overuse injuries include lateral and medial tendinopathies, ulna collateral ligament injury and Valgus Extension Overload (VEO).

In Europe, where there is less dominance of pitching sports, other common sporting injuries to the elbow are seen (Table 10.1) and it should be noted that the patterns of injuries seen in adolescents differ from those seen in adults [6, 7].

To compensate for the physical forces placed on the structures, an athlete's upper limb develops marked physical adaptations [6, 8].

10.2 Physical Adaptations to Overhead Activities

Adaptations in range of motion, ligamentous laxity and muscular compensation are seen in the throwing limb of athletes, compared with the contra-lateral upper limb, which means between sides comparisons may not be adequate when restoring an athlete back to their pre-injury baseline [7, 8].

A body of evidence shows the presence of medial elbow laxity, significant elbow flexion contractures and a significant decrease in wrist flexibility in the dominant arm of overhead athletes [9, 10]. There is also an increased strength profile for the dominant arm in the glenohumeral joint internal rotators, elbow, wrist and forearm muscles, seen in tennis players, baseball pitchers and javelin throwers [11–17].

However, it should be noted that muscle group strength ratios are sport specific. In some overhead activities such as volleyball and tennis, high elbow extensor to flexor ratios are seen [17], whereas in activities such as judo, there is an almost equal ratio of elbow extensors to flexors [18]. This should be borne in mind when designing individual rehabilitation programmes.

10.3 General Rehabilitation

The aim of rehabilitation is to expose healing tissues to appropriate stress and avoid the adverse changes to tissue biomechanics and morphology seen after prolonged immobilisation.

According to Wilk et al. [7], rehabilitation following elbow injury or surgery (Table 10.2) follows a sequential, well defined approach, where phases overlap to ensure the athlete returns to their previous functional level as quickly and safely as possible. The approach is based on best current available evidence, adapted to each individual and their respective sport. Progression through a rehabilitation regimen should be based on targets rather than time. Time points should be used as a guide only.

10.4 Acute Phase

The first phase is the immediate motion phase, where the goals are to reduce the deleterious effects of immobilisation, to re-establish motion, decrease pain, decrease inflammation and retard muscle atrophy [7, 19].

Table 10.2 Example guidelines for progression of rehabilitation

Surgical procedure	Early stage	Intermediate stage	Late stage	Return to sport
Collateral ligament reconstruction	Immediately post op	Gradual progression between weeks 2–6	Week 6+ Week 8+ for Plyometrics	From Week 12
Distal biceps repair with endobutton	Immediately post op, within safe ROM	Weeks 2–12	Week 12	12+ weeks
Long flexor/extensor tendon origin repair	Immediately post op	Weeks 3–8	Week 8	Week 12

Communication with the surgeon is essential, to ensure a good understanding of the integrity of the repair. Timescales are approximate guidelines only.

For some specific surgery, if AROM is to be restricted to allow tissue healing, it is beneficial to have a 'safe zone' as established by the surgeon prior to closure. This can be utilised to progress rehabilitation within the safe zone without putting the repair at risk.

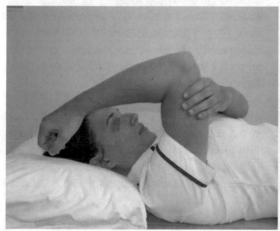 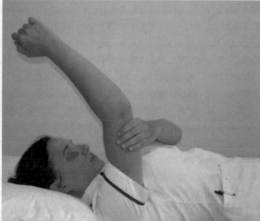

Fig. 10.1 Overhead pictures

Movement is initiated as soon as it is safely possible, as progressive mechanical loading is more likely to restore morphological characteristics of tissues, such as capsuloligamentous, osteochondral and muscular structures [20, 21]. Animal models have demonstrated that loading upregulates genetic expression for key proteins associated with tissue healing [20–22]. Clinical studies have demonstrated that immediate elbow mobilisation, even post-dislocation, results in less loss of motion with no apparent increase in instability [23]. The safe arc of motion is dictated by healing constraints of soft tissues as well as the specific pathology or surgery [7].

Mobilisation exercises are performed, in this protected range, as defined by surgery/injury, frequently throughout the day, for all planes of elbow, forearm, and wrist motion. There should

be a bias towards active mobilisation, as muscular activation stabilises the elbow, when compared with passive mobilisation alone [24]. The elbow joint is especially prone to flexion contractures, therefore, establishing full pre-injury extension, as early as possible, is a primary goal.

The overhead position described by Wolff and Hotchkiss [25] is the optimal mobilisation position to achieve this goal (Fig. 10.1).

This position has been demonstrated to maximise elbow stability, by minimising ulno-humeral distraction [26]. Distraction is most marked with the arm hanging dependent by the side, especially when wearing a cast or hinged elbow brace, and therefore, this position should be avoided for exercises. The overhead position also has the added benefit of minimising biceps EMG activity seen clinically in the painful, stiff elbow [27], and enhances triceps activity, thereby maximising elbow extension range. This position is suitable for the majority of individuals with conservatively managed elbow pathology. However, it is only suitable for post-operative patients, where a triceps sparing approach has been taken.

Initially, active assisted flexion/extension is performed with the contralateral upper limb providing support where needed. The forearm position during this exercise, is dependent on any capsule-ligamentous structures that need protecting. With lateral compartment lesions, the forearm is placed in pronation, whereby passive tension in the common extensor origin contributes to lateral stability. Supination is the optimal position for medial compartment lesions [24]. As soon as comfort allows, the exercises are progressed to active movements without assistance.

It is of great importance that any exercise or alternative techniques used in this stage produce minimal pain, as neuropeptides such as Substance P, involved in pain transmission, can be associated with increased myofibroblastic activity [28]. This is seen in individuals with contracted elbow capsules, a common complication seen after elbow trauma or surgery. Supplemental manual therapy may also be used in the early phase to modulate pain, by stimulating type I/II articular receptors [7]. In elbow tendinopathy, mobilisations with movements can be applied, where they have a demonstrable effect on decreasing pain on symptomatic activities such as grip [29].

During the acute phase, focus is also placed on voluntary activation of muscles and reducing muscular atrophy. Isometric exercises of the major elbow, forearm and wrist muscle groups are performed, which have been shown place no additional strain on healing ligamentous grafts [30]. Contractions are performed at the common flexor pronator group and the common extensor group, which are secondary stabilisers of the medial and lateral compartments, respectively [31]. The dynamic stabilisers, including triceps, biceps and anconeus, that produce compression at the elbow are also targeted [31]. The anconeus appears from both EMG and anatomical studies to be a lateral elbow stabiliser, co-apting the ulna

to the humerus, reducing postero-lateral rotatory displacement [32–34], and can be facilitated isometrically even when the elbow is immobilised in a plaster cast or splint.

Isometric contractions also have the additional benefit of reducing pain, via a generalised, centrally induced, pain inhibitory response. The magnitude of this effect increases with contractions of longer durations, of moderate or above intensity (40–50% MVC) and is not constrained to the exercising limb [35–40].

If the patient has had surgery, consideration must be given to the integrity of the musculo-tendinous units in order to guide early resistance work [41]. This requires good communication between the surgeon and therapist about the surgical approach employed, structures injured, divided and repaired.

Shoulder isometric work may be performed with caution with resistance applied proximal to the elbow. However, care should be taken with positions of extreme glenohumeral external rotation, as they produce a valgus moment at the elbow, possibly compromising vulnerable tissues [41].

10.5 Intermediate Stage

This is commenced when the following is achieved, a return to pre-injury range, with minimal pain and tenderness and good strength of elbow and forearm musculature [7], usually at 4–6 weeks post-injury/surgery.

Elbow extension and forearm pronation is of particular importance for effective performance in throwing sports [7, 19]. Local strengthening exercises are progressed to isotonic contractions, beginning with concentric work, then eccentric work, with emphasis placed on the secondary stabilisers [7] (Fig. 10.2).

With medial compartment symptoms, emphasis should be placed on the flexor pronator mass, especially flexor carpi ulnaris, which anatomical and EMG studies have been shown to contribute to valgus stability, by reducing forces placed on ulnar collateral ligament, during throwing [42–44]. With tendinopathy, the key goal is improving

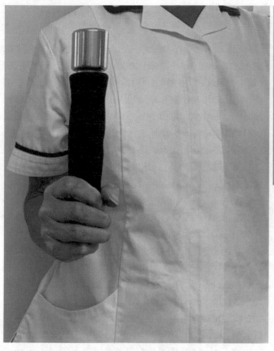
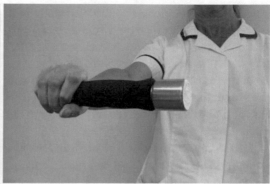

Fig. 10.2 Pro/supination with weighted bar

the capacity of the tendon and muscle to manage load. Several strengthening options exist, as well as heavy slow resistance work, all sharing a common goal of gradually increasing load, whilst carefully monitoring pain. This approach for tendinopathy has been supported by clinical trials, with long-term benefits seen compared with pharmacological and electrotherapy interventions [45–47]. Counterforce bracing is only useful in individuals where it demonstrably reduces pain or improves grip, and is only worn during pain provoking activities [48].

Emphasis is also placed on exercises improving endurance and neuro-muscular control of the elbow complex [7, 19, 49]. Loss of kinaesthetic awareness of upper extremities can occur post-injury, and has been shown to decrease proprioceptive accuracy in throwers [50–53]. Proprioceptive neuromuscular facilitation, rhythmic stabilisation drills and open and closed kinetic chain activities, which promote co-contraction and mimic functional positions with joint approximation, are now implemented [7]. Studies show a decrease in neuro muscular con-

trol, kinaesthetic detection strength and throwing accuracy is associated with muscular fatigue, therefore exercises, including multiple sets [8], to promote endurance are a key component of this stage.

Shoulder flexibility is also addressed at this stage, as loss of total shoulder rotational range or gleno-humeral internal rotation deficit (GIRD) has been shown to place strain on medial elbow structures during throwing [54]. Postero-inferior gleno-humeral capsular tightening and shrinkage, along with adaptive humeral head changes are well-documented problems in long-term throwers [54–56]. For this group, stretches such as a sleeper stretch are thought to be effective in addressing the capsular tightness [57]. Care should be taken with stretches at extremes of glenohumeral external rotation, as mentioned previously. It is also important not to apply this to all individuals with elbow injury or pathology. It must be considered that the GIRD may be a problem of control, rather than of capsular origin [57–59]. For this group stretching may not be as effective, and the problem should be addressed by performing eccentric and concentric rotator cuff exercises through range [57]. It is essential that the individual is carefully assessed to ensure that any deficit is managed appropriately. Therefore a comprehensive assessment of the shoulder and the scapula should be undertaken, as scapula dysfunction prevents optimum energy transfer in the upper limb.

Gleno-humeral rotational strength and scapula strength is addressed during this phase, and are incorporated in the Throwers 10 strengthening programme [60]. This has been designed, from EMG evidence, to illicit muscular activity most needed to provide upper limb dynamic stability, and has been demonstrated to increase throwing velocity, following a 6 week programme [8, 61, 62]. Attention should be paid to global upper limb strengthening, even with elbow tendinopathy, as previous studies have shown global weakness, affecting all major shoulder groups, and the triceps, with this condition 67, probably due to pain inhibition and disuse [63].

It is vital not only to concentrate on the upper limb, but on the whole kinetic chain at this stage in rehabilitation, the kinetic chain being a specific sequence of movement which allows efficient accomplishment of a task. Injuries or adaptations in remote areas of the chain can cause problems not only locally, but also distally, as joints such as the elbow compensate for lack of force production and energy delivery through more proximal links [7, 64].

Kibler and Chandler calculated a 20% reduction in kinetic energy delivered from the hip and trunk to the upper limb, require a 34% increase in rotational velocity of the arm, to impart the same amount of force to the hand [65]. Hannon's study 70 has shown a link between lower limb balance deficits in throwers with medial elbow ligament injuries, compared with healthy controls [66]. These balance deficits disappear following a 3 month throwers rehab programme including the trunk and the lower limb. Therefore, in this early stage, whilst the elbow is recovering, leg and trunk exercises involving sport specific activation patterns can be initiated, so that the base of the kinetic chain is ready for the next phase, late stage rehabilitation.

10.6 Late Stage Rehabilitation

The ultimate aim of late stage rehabilitation' is to prepare the individual for a return to sport with confidence, and with as minimal risk of injury as possible. In order to achieve this, full concentric and eccentric strength, power, endurance, and control must be achieved throughout the upper quadrant and kinetic chain.

Late stage rehabilitation can be commenced when the individual has minimal or no pain on palpation, near full active range of movement, and 70% of their predicted (or previously recorded) strength [7]. It is essential that the stage of healing is considered specifically for the injured tissue type, and that the tissue involved is theoretically considered to have achieved a sufficient degree of repair or stability. Depending on the particular tissue type and the individual, it is suggested that progression to late stage rehabilitation will commence between 7 and 12 weeks post injury or surgery.

Late stage rehabilitation will continue until the individual successfully returns to sport. It should be remembered that to return an athlete to competition may take up to 12 months, with athletes throwing for short periods of time at 3 months post-op [41]. It should include an exercise programme with a gradual increase in resistance, an increase in muscle work through a wider range of movement, and a steady increase in lever length. It should gradually become more dynamic, with a reduction in predictability, and an increase in weight bearing exercise and activities. This stage should also commence plyometric exercise and controlled impact work.

At this stage basic range of motion ought to have been achieved. It is important to concentrate on sports specific functional patterns of movement, and on the principles of proprioceptive, neuromuscular facilitation (PNF) and motor learning [67]. This can be achieved by exaggerating movement patterns performed during the specific sport [7].

It is vital to address any deficits or ongoing problems in terms of ROM. For a lack of elbow extension and or flexion, it is important to go back to the basics discussed in the previous stages to regain elbow range.

Strengthening should follow the principles described above with regards to functional and sport specific patterns of movement. Load should be increased gradually, as should the length of lever. Therapists should design an exercise programme specific to the individual's sport. Alternatively an established programme such as the 'Advanced Thrower's Ten' should be initiated [68].

Strengthening should address the entire upper quadrant, and ought to progress strengthening exercises for the rotator cuff, and scapula, already started in the intermediate phase [69–72]. Exercise should include both concentric and eccentric work through the full available range [7, 9]. Again, it is essential to consider sport specific eccentric control, for example the deceleration phase in throwing 8. During deceleration there is a marked biceps and brachialis activity, decelerating the rapidly extending elbow and pronating forearm, which need addressing during this stage.

Strengthening exercises should be performed in a dynamic manner incorporating the full kinetic chain mentioned previously, and should address proximal stability as part of the chain [72]. The strengthening programme should be progressed by reducing positions of stability [73]. An example of progression of an exercise would be that of a tennis forehand movement with an exercise band; this would be initiated with a step forward, to stepping in different directions, to lunges, whilst altering the position of the upper limb (in terms of degrees of shoulder abduction +/− flexion), increasing the lever length (elbow flexion/ extension), to ultimately increasing the speed of lunge, and upper limb movement, and increasing the load. Each element should be progressed slowly, and only one component increased at a time to avoid overload or injury. Progression could also be made by initially hitting a low compression ball, seen in mini tennis, to then move on to a regular tennis ball.

The therapist should carefully consider the sport for which they are rehabilitating and tailor the strengthening programme accordingly, especially muscle group ratios, as discussed previously. For example in disciplines such as the

bars in gymnastics, it is essential that a strengthening programme includes weight bearing exercises such as a progression to handstand work. All strengthening programmes should start with low resistance and high repetitions and progress slowly [73].

10.6.1 Plyometrics

Plyometrics are commonly used in late stage rehabilitation to improve the power and neuromuscular control of a limb. They are designed to activate the stretch-shortening cycle and increase the excitability of the neurological receptors to improve the reactivity of the neuromuscular system [14, 15]. The stretch of the musculo-tendinous unit immediately followed by shortening is key to the concept of plyometric exercise, and this stretch-shortening cycle enhances the ability of the musculo-tendinous unit to produce maximum force in the shortest time [74]. They are commonly used to increase strength and power, and are considered to be the bridge between pure power and sports related speed, and ultimately thought to enhance athletic performance [74, 75]. In practice plyometric exercises mimic the dynamic and explosive characteristics of many sports.

A plyometric programme should be structured and tailored to the individual.

Example of an plyometric program

Week	
1	Two handed throws and wrist flips Low impact ball progress to standard ball
2	One handed throws and wrist flips Standard ball progressing to heavy ball
3	Reduce predictability Trampet throws Med progressing to heavy ball One progressing to two handed
4	Weight bearing plyometrics Trampet press ups—add in clap Bosu ball press up/bounce/clap

In order for an exercise to be deemed plyometric it is essential that the change in muscle recruitment (point of impact) is sudden. This should mimic the sport for which you are rehabilitating. For example when playing squash, the ball makes contact with the racquet for less than 1 second. Therefore plyometric training should reflect this. Throwing activities involving the shoulder and elbow should commence with two handed low load, high repetition, predictable plyometrics (Fig. 10.3), and should progress to one handed, unpredictable (Fig. 10.4), dynamic plyometrics, on a stable platform, but can ultimately end on an unstable platform, e.g. gym ball, or wobble board. Other examples of plyometric activities localised to forearm flexors include wrist flips and snaps [7].

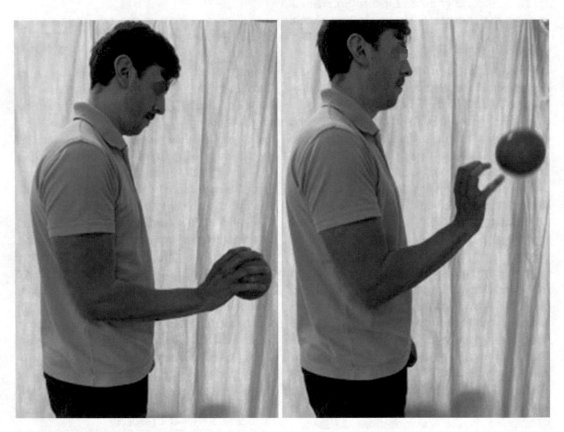

Fig. 10.3 Wrist flips and snaps

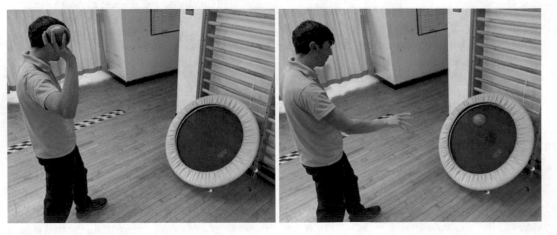

Fig. 10.4 Plyometric throw

10.6.2 Impact Work

For individuals who wish to return to contact sports e.g. rugby, it is vital to address impact work at this stage. Previous studies have shown that increased muscle activation patterns of the elbow and wrist during forward falls, increase the transition of force shock waves through the forearm [76]. With practice, individuals can select the upper extremity posture, allowing the athlete to minimise the effects of impact. Lo showed that practising 5–10 repetitions of forward falls, result in decreased impact forces in the upper limb, during subsequent falls, for the following 2 months [77].

10.6.3 Return to Sport

It is essential that the return to sport phase is fully addressed, failure to do so may put the individual at risk of injury or reduce their performance. Prior to returning to sport the individual must be painfree, with no tenderness, have adequate dynamic stability, have completed a satisfactory isokinetic test, and have been assessed on their ability to perform sports specific drills [73, 78].

Interval sports programmes (ISP) are widely accepted as an appropriate method of training a sports person for their return to sport. The principle of an ISP involves a graduated return to sport specific activities following injury or surgery [59, 73, 78]. ISPs should be designed on an individual basis, and should include, specific sport related activities involving the full kinetic chain, a gradual progression of applied forces, a comprehensive warm-up, and correct biomechanical alignment and technique [78]. Examples of ISPs have been published, including ISPs for throwers, golf, and racquet sports, and are widely available.

Example of Tennis ISP

Week	Effort	FH	BH	Serves	Rest	Play	Repeat
1	50% Shots	12–15	7–10	0	10 min	Nil	×2
2	75% Shots	25–30	15–25	0	10 min	Nil	×2
3	75% Shots 50% Serves	30	25–30	10–15	10 min	Nil	×2–3
4	100% Shots 75% Serves	30	30	10	10 min	3 games Set 1.5 sets	×2
		After rest and play, reduce shots					
		10	10	5			
5	100% Shots 75% Serves	30–20	30–20	30–15	10 min	Set 1.5 Sets	×2
6	100% Shots 100% Serves	30	30	30	10 min	1.5 sets	×2
NB	Play only performed once daily, repeat training pre and post play. Return to full play after week 6						

Adapted from Reinold et al. [78]

The duration of the ISP should be specific to the individual, and will vary dependent on the sport person's injury, skill level and goals. Towards completion of the ISP, a plan for the start of full participation in sport ought to be made. This should include an adequate warm-up which should include the full kinetic chain. A sport specific warm-up that has been demonstrated to activate appropriate musculature is ideal, for example an exercise band programme for throwers [79]. The game or competition should be followed by an appropriate cool down, and ongoing exercise programme to prevent further injury.

Q&A

Q1: What is the primary goal of the acute phase of rehabilitation?

The goal of acute phase rehabilitation are to reduce the deleterious effects of immobilisation, to re-establish motion, decrease pain, decrease inflammation and retard muscle atrophy.

Q2: What is the optimal position for early mobilisation of the elbow?

The overhead position described by Wolff and Hotchkiss is the optimal mobilisation position for early mobilisation as it maximises elbow stability, minimises biceps activity and enhances triceps activity, thereby maximising elbow extension range.

Q3: Why should the injured elbow not be compared to the contralateral elbow in sports persons.

Many sports require very different function of each limb and equivalence should not be expected.

Q4: What is the role of the kinetic chain?

The kinetic chain can be used synchronously to provide power to the upper limb. Injuries or adaptations in remote areas of the kinetic chain can cause problems as the elbow compensates for lack of force production and energy delivery through more proximal parts of the chain. A 20% reduction in kinetic energy delivered from the hip and trunk to the upper limb, require a 34% increase in rotational velocity of the arm, to impart the same amount of force to the hand. Therefore, whilst the elbow is recovering, leg and trunk exercises involving sport specific activation patterns can be initiated, so that the base of the kinetic chain provides stable support to upper limb function.

Q5: Give an example of a plyometric exercise.

Wrist flips and snaps are examples of plyometric exercises. In order for an exercise to be deemed plyometric it is essential that the change in muscle recruitment (point of impact) is sudden. Plyometrics are commonly used in late stage rehabilitation to mimic the dynamic and explosive characteristics of many sports. A plyometric programme should be structured and tailored to the individual.

References

1. Conte S, Requa RK, Garrick JG. Disability days in major league baseball. Am J Sports Med. 2001;29(4):431–6.
2. Posner M, Cameron KL, Wolf JM, Belmont PJ Jr, Owens BD. Epidemiology of Major League Baseball injuries. Am J Sports Med. 2011;39(8):1676–80.
3. Priest JD. Tennis elbow. The syndrome and a study of average players. Minn Med. 1976;59(6):367–71.
4. Wilson FD, Andrews JR, Blackburn TA, Mccluskey G. Valgus extension overload in the pitching elbow. Am J Sports Med. 1983;11(2):83–8.
5. Cain EL, Dugas JR, Wolf RS, Andrews JR. Elbow injuries in throwing athletes a current concepts review. Am J Sports Med. 2003;31(4):621–35.
6. Crotin RL, Ramsey DK. Injury prevention for throwing athletes Part I: Baseball bat training to enhance medial elbow dynamic stability. Strength Cond J. 2012;34(2):79–85.
7. Wilk KE, Macrina LC, Cain EL, Dugas JR, Andrews JR. Rehabilitation of the overhead athlete's elbow. Sports Health. 2012;4(5):404–14.
8. Ellenbecker TS, Nirschl R, Renstrom P. Current concepts in examination and treatment of elbow tendon injury. Sports Health. 2012;1941738112464761.
9. Ellenbecker TS, Mattalino AJ, Elam EA, Caplinger RA. Medial elbow joint laxity in professional baseball pitchers: a bilateral comparison using stress radiography. Am J Sports Med. 1998;26(3):420–4.
10. Wright RW, Steger-May K, Wasserlauf BL, O'Neal ME, Weinberg BW, Paletta GA. Elbow range of motion in professional baseball pitchers. Am J Sports Med. 2006;34(2):190–3.
11. Ellenbecker TS, Roetert EP, Riewald S. Isokinetic profile of wrist and forearm strength in elite female junior tennis players. Br J Sports Med. 2006;40(5):411–4.
12. Kovacs MS, Ellenbecker TS. A performance evaluation of the tennis serve: implications for strength, speed, power, and flexibility training. Strength Cond J. 2011;33(4):22–30.
13. Laudner KG, Wilson JT, Meister K. Elbow isokinetic strength characteristics among collegiate baseball players. Phys Ther Sport. 2012;13(2):97–100.
14. Wilk KE, Arrigo C, Andrews JR. Rehabilitation of the elbow in the throwing athlete. J Orthop Sports Phys Ther. 1993a;17(6):30.
15. Wilk KE, Voight ML, Keirns MA, Gambetta V, Andrews JR, Dillman CJ. Stretch-shortening drills for the upper extremities: theory and clinical application. J Orthop Sports Phys Ther. 1993b;17(5):225–39.
16. Ellenbecker TS. A total arm strength isokinetic profile of highly skilled tennis players. Isokinet Exerc Sci. 1991;1(1):9–21.
17. Ellenbecker TS, Roetert EP. Isokinetic profile of elbow flexion and extension strength in elite junior tennis players. J Orthop Sports Phys Ther. 2003;33(2):79–84.
18. Ruivo R, Pezarat-Correia P, Carita AI. Elbow and shoulder muscles strength profile in judo athletes. Isokinet Exerc Sci. 2012;20(1):41–5.
19. Wilk KE, Reinold MM, Andrews JR. Rehabilitation of the thrower's elbow. Clin Sports Med. 2004;23(4):765–801.
20. Bring DKI, Reno C, Renstrom P, Salo P, Hart DA, Ackermann PW. Joint immobilization reduces the expression of sensory neuropeptide receptors and impairs healing after tendon rupture in a rat model. J Orthop Res. 2009;27(2):274–80.

21. Martinez DA, Vailas AC, Vanderby JR, Grindeland RE. Temporal extracellular matrix adaptations in ligament during wound healing and hindlimb unloading. Am J Phys Regul Integr Comp Phys. 2007;293(4):R1552–60.

22. Eliasson P, Andersson T, Aspenberg P. Rat Achilles tendon healing: mechanical loading and gene expression. J Appl Physiol. 2009;107(2):399–407.

23. Ross G, McDevitt ER, Chronister R, Ove PN. Treatment of simple elbow dislocation using an immediate motion protocol. Am J Sports Med. 1999;27(3):308–11.

24. Armstrong AD, Dunning CE, Faber KJ, Duck TR, Johnson JA, King GJ. Rehabilitation of the medial collateral ligament-deficient elbow: an in vitro biomechanical study. J Hand Surg. 2000;25(6):1051–7.

25. Wolff AL, Hotchkiss RN. Lateral elbow instability: nonoperative, operative, and postoperative management. J Hand Ther. 2006;19(2):238–44.

26. Lee AT, Schrumpf MA, Choi D, Meyers KN, Patel R, Wright TM, Daluiski A. The influence of gravity on the unstable elbow. J Shoulder Elb Surg. 2013;22(1):81–7.

27. Page C, Backus SI, Lenhoff MW. Electromyographic activity in stiff and normal elbows during elbow flexion and extension. J Hand Ther. 2003;16(1):5–11.

28. Monument MJ, Hart DA, Salo PT, Befus AD, Hildebrand KA. Posttraumatic elbow contractures: targeting neuroinflammatory fibrogenic mechanisms. J Orthop Sci. 2013;18(6):869–77.

29. Bisset L, Coombes B, Vicenzino B. Tennis elbow. BMJ Clin Evid. 2011 Jun 27;2011:1117. PMID: 21708051; PMCID: PMC3217754.

30. Bernas GA, Thiele RAR, Kinnaman KA, Hughes RE, Miller BS, Carpenter JE. Defining safe rehabilitation for ulnar collateral ligament reconstruction of the elbow: a biomechanical study. Am J Sports Med. 2009;37(12):2392–400.

31. O'Driscoll SW, Jupiter JB, King GJ, Hotchkiss RN, Morrey BF. The unstable elbow. J Bone Joint Surg. 2000;82(5):724.

32. Basmajian JV, Griffin W Jr. Function of anconeus muscle an electromyographic study. J Bone Joint Surg. 1972;54(8):1712–4.

33. Bergin MJG, Vicenzino B, Hodges PW. Functional differences between anatomical regions of the anconeus muscle in humans. J Electromyogr Kinesiol. 2013;236:1391–7.

34. Molinier F, Laffosse JM, Bouali O, Tricoire JL, Moscovici J. The anconeus, an active lateral ligament of the elbow: new anatomical arguments. Surg Radiol Anat. 2011;33(7):617–21.

35. Koltyn KF, Umeda M. Contralateral attenuation of pain after short-duration submaximal isometric exercise. J Pain. 2007;8(11):887–92.

36. Kosek E, Ekholm J. Modulation of pressure pain thresholds during and following isometric contraction. Pain. 1995;61(3):481–6.

37. Kosek E, Lundberg L. Segmental and plurisegmental modulation of pressure pain thresholds during static muscle contractions in healthy individuals. Eur J Pain. 2003;7(3):251–8.

38. Lannersten L, Kosek E. Dysfunction of endogenous pain inhibition during exercise with painful muscles in patients with shoulder myalgia and fibromyalgia. Pain. 2010;151(1):77–86.

39. Misra G, Paris TA, Archer DB, Coombes SA. Dose-response effect of isometric force production on the perception of pain. PLoS One. 2014;9(2):e88105.

40. Staud R, Robinson ME, Price DD. Isometric exercise has opposite effects on central pain mechanisms in fibromyalgia patients compared to normal controls. Pain. 2005;118(1):176–84.

41. Ellenbecker TS, Wilk KE, Altchek DW, Andrews JR. Current concepts in rehabilitation following ulnar collateral ligament reconstruction. Sports Health. 2009;1(4):301–13.

42. Lin F. Muscle contribution to elbow joint valgus stability. J Shoulder Elb Surg. 2007;16(6):795–802.

43. Park MC, Ahmad CS. Dynamic contributions of the flexor-pronator mass to elbow valgus stability. J Bone Joint Surg. 2004;86(10):2268–74.

44. Perry J, Jobe FW. Functional anatomy of the flexor pronator muscle group in relation to the medial collateral ligament of the elbow. Am J Sports Med. 1995;23(2):245–50.

45. Pienimäki TT, Tarvainen TK, Siira PT, Vanharanta H. Progressive strengthening and stretching exercises and ultrasound for chronic lateral epicondylitis. Physiotherapy. 1996;82(9):522–30.

46. Stasinopoulos D, Stasinopoulou K, Johnson MI. An exercise programme for the management of lateral elbow tendinopathy. Br J Sports Med. 2005;39(12):944–7.

47. Svernlöv B, Adolfsson L. Non-operative treatment regime including eccentric training for lateral humeral epicondylalgia. Scand J Med Sci Sports. 2001;11(6):328–34.

48. Ng G. The effects of forearm brace tension on neuromuscular performance in subjects with lateral humeral epicondylosis: a review. Int Sport Med J. 2005;6(2):124. Review article. Elbow Injuries in Sport: Part 2: The Biomechanics of the Elbow in Sport.

49. Fusaro I, Orsini S, Kantar SS, Sforza T, Benedetti MG, Bettelli G, Rotini R. Elbow rehabilitation in traumatic pathology. Musculoskelet Surg. 2014;98(1):95–102.

50. Carpenter JE, Blasier RB, Pellizzon GG. The effects of muscle fatigue on shoulder joint position sense. Am J Sports Med. 1998;26(2):262–5.

51. Guskiewicz KM, Schneider RA, Prentice WE. Proprioception and neuromuscular control of the shoulder after muscle fatigue. J Athl Train. 1999;34(4):362.

52. Myers JB, Ju YY, Hwang JH, McMahon PJ, Rodosky MW, Lephart SM. Reflexive muscle activation alterations in shoulders with anterior glenohumeral instability. Am J Sports Med. 2004;32(4):1013–21.

53. Voight ML, Hardin JA, Blackburn TA, Tippett S, Canner GC. The effects of muscle fatigue on and the relationship of arm dominance to shoulder proprioception. J Orthop Sports Phys Ther. 1996;23(6):348–52.

54. Shanley E, Rauh MJ, Michener LA, Ellenbecker TS, Garrison JC, Thigpen CA. Shoulder range of motion

measures as risk factors for shoulder and elbow injuries in high school softball and baseball players. Am J Sports Med. 2011;39(9):1997–2006.

55. Grossman MG, Tibone JE, McGary MH, Schneider DJ, Veneziani S, Lee TQ. A Cadaveric model of the throwing shoulder: a possible etiology of superior labrum anterior to posterior lesions. J Bone Joint Surg Am. 2005;87(4):824–31.

56. Tokish JM, Curtin MS, Young-Kyu K, Hawkins RJ, Torry MR. Glenohumeral internal rotation deficit in the asymptomaticprofessional pitcher and its relationship to humeral retroversion. J Sports Sci Med. 2008;7:78–83.

57. Jaggi A, Lambert S. Rehabilitation for shoulder instability. Br J Sports Med. 2010;44:333–40.

58. Boettcher CE, Cathers I, Ginn KA. The role of shoulder muscles is task specific. J Sci Med Sport. 2010;13(6):651–6.

59. Ellenbecker T, Cools A. Rehabilitation of shoulder impingement syndrome and rotator cuff injuries: an evidence based review. Br J Sports Med. 2010;44:319–27.

60. Wilk KE, Obma P, Simpson CD, Cain EL, Dugas J, Andrews JR. Shoulder injuries in the overhead athlete. J Orthopaed Sports Phys Ther. 2009;39(2):38–54.

61. Reinold MM, Wilk KE, Fleisig GS, Zheng N, Barrentine SW, Chmielewski T, Cody RC, Jameson GG, Andrews JR. Electromyographic analysis of the rotator cuff and deltoid musculature during common shoulder external rotation exercises. J Orthop Sports Phys Ther. 2004;34(7):385–94.

62. Reinold MM, Macrina LC, Wilk KE, Fleisig GS, Dun S, Barrentine SW, Andrews JR. Electromyographic analysis of the supraspinatus and deltoid muscles during 3 common rehabilitation exercises. J Athl Train. 2007;42(4):464–9.

63. Alizadehkhaiyat O, Fisher AC, Kemp GJ, Vishwanathan K, Frostick SP. Upper limb muscle imbalance in tennis elbow: a functional and electromyographic assessment. J Orthop Res. 2007;25(12):1651–7.

64. Seroyer ST, Nho SJ, Bach BR, Bush-Joseph CA, Nicholson GP, Romeo AA. The kinetic chain in overhand pitching: its potential role for performance enhancement and injury prevention. Sports Health. 2010;2(2):135–46.

65. Kibler WB, Chandler J. Baseball and tennis. In: Griffin LY, editor. Rehabilitation of the injured knee. St. Louis, MO: Mosby; 1995. p. 219–26.

66. Hannon J, Garrison JC, Conway J. Lower extremity balance is improved at time of return to throwing in baseball players after an ulnar collateral ligament reconstruction when compared to pre-operative measurements. Int J Sports Phys Ther. 2014;9(3):356.

67. Cook G, Burton L, Hoogenboom BJ, Voight M. Functional movement screening: the use of fundamental movements as an assessment of function-part 1. Int J Sports Phys Ther. 2014 Jun 1;9(3).

68. Wilk KE, Yenchak AJ, Arrigo CA, Andrews JR. The Advanced Throwers Ten Exercise Program: a new exercise series for enhanced dynamic shoulder control in the overhead throwing athlete. Phys Sportsmed. 2011;39(4):90–7.

69. Ballantyne BT, O'Hare SJ, Paschall JL, Pavia-Smith MM, Pitz AM, Gillon JF, Soderberg GL. Electromyographic activity of selected shoulder muscles in commonly used therapeutic exercises. Phys Ther. 1993;73(10):668–77.

70. Ekstrom RA, Donatelli RA, Soderberg GL. Surface electromyographic analysis of exercises for the trapezius and serratus anterior muscles. J Orthop Sports Phys Ther. 2003;33(5):247–58.

71. Kim H, Lee Y, Shin I, Kim K, Moon J. Effects of 8 weeks' specific physical training on the rotator cuff muscle strength and technique of javelin throwers. J Phys Ther Sci. 2014;26(10):1553–6.

72. Kibler WB, Wilkes T, Sciascia A. Mechanics and pathomechanics in the overhead athlete. Clin Sports Med. 2013;32(4):637–51.

73. Ellenbecker TS, Nirschl R, Renstrom P. Current concepts in examination and treatment of elbow tendon injury. Sports Health. 2013;5(2):186–94.

74. Chmielewski TL, Myer GD, Kauffman D, Tillman SM. Plyometric exercise in the rehabilitation of athletes: physiological responses and clinical application. J Orthop Sports Phys Ther. 2006;36(5):308–19.

75. Schulte-Edelmann JA, Davies GJ, Kernozek TW, Gerberding ED. The effects of plyometric training of the posterior shoulder and elbow. J Strength Cond Res. 2005;19(1):129–34.

76. Burkhart TA, Andrews DM. Kinematics, kinetics and muscle activation patterns of the upper extremity during simulated forward falls. J Electromyogr Kinesiol. 2013;23(3):688–95.

77. Lo J, McCabe GN, DeGoede KM, Okuizumi H, Ashton-Miller JA. On reducing hand impact force in forward falls: results of a brief intervention in young males. Clin Biomech. 2003;18(8):730–6.

78. Reinold MM, Wilk KE, Reed J, Crenshaw K, Andrews JR. Interval sport programs: guidelines for baseball, tennis, and golf. J Orthop Sports Phys Ther. 2002;32(6):293–8.

79. Myers JB, Pasquale MR, Laudner KG, Sell TC, Bradley JP, Lephart SM. On-the-field resistance-tubing exercises for throwers: an electromyographic analysis. J Athletic Train. 2005 Jan;40(1):15.

Index

A. C. Watts et al. (eds.), *Sports Injuries of the Elbow*, https://doi.org/10.1007/978-3-030-52379-4

Printed in the United States
by Baker & Taylor Publisher Services